True Jo

From Within

The Englishman
with Fibromyalgia

Life Before & Life Now

Shayne E Town

True Journey From Within The Englishman With Fibromyalgia
Life Before & Life Now © Shayne E Town 2016

Pulbished by Lilly Pilly Publishing
www.lillypillypublishing.com

Lilly Pilly
Publishing

Fibromyalgia ribbon image © Claire Wallace, 2016
Scroll by 123rf
Copyright for individual stories remains with the authors.

ISBN: 978-0-9945366-0-0 (paperback)

I would like to dedicate this book to my dear Mum & Dad,
who have always stood by my side in times of need,
and who have supported me throughout.

This book is also dedicated to the millions of people
who are constantly battling with fibromyalgia everyday,
just to try and find a little bit of peace in their lives.

Acknowledgements

A special thank you to Michelle Cardno Llb (Hons) for her opening foreword.

A special thank you to Janet Ward for overseeing the book and her contributions.

A special thank you to all who have contributed their stories:
Ella Cooper, Connie Thompson, Jules Allen, Tracey Crookes, Robert Fraser, Linda Morris Ellard, Beth Urmston, Ian Hydon, Cheryl Gomery, Esther Whitwam, Chelle Priestley, Pam Wooller, Andrea Raso and Donna Turner.

Note to the Reader

Thank you for purchasing this book. I hope the information contained will give you a little better understanding of fibromyalgia and the possibilities of moving forward. This book is my own personal journey and is for general informational purposes only. It is not intended to replace any medical advice given by your doctor. If you feel you have any signs and symptoms of fibromyalgia please consult with your own doctor if you need medical attention.

Useful addresses (UK) and all internet addresses including email addresses were correct at time of going to press.

The royalties made from this book will all go to fund "*Fibroduck Foundation*" for research to help find a much needed cure.

Foreword

This is an easy to read and resourceful account from the very beginning of Shayne's journey. It is suitable for health care professionals and sufferers who are affected by fibromyalgia and the various complex symptoms associated with the condition.

Having known Shayne for a number of years, I have had the great pleasure in writing this foreword for his book. It outlines how the condition has affected his life and has spurned him on to raise awareness and help others. Fibromyalgia is a seriously misunderstood condition which is affecting millions of people around the world, and numbers continue to rise at an alarming rate each year. Often sufferers struggle to cope with the complexities of it, and this book gives a heartfelt account and insight into the life of someone who has proactively gained much knowledge through research and determination to help fellow sufferers.

At *Fightback4Justice* we speak to people who suffer with this same condition on a day to day basis, often helping them fill out various forms and helping them with appeals when health care professionals trivialise the effects of fibromyalgia. The stress can, in turn aggravate their symptoms, leaving them more overwhelmed and alone.

This book covers fibromyalgia from an in-depth, personal insight, of living and managing this condition. Shayne uses his own words to describe exactly how fibromyalgia has disrupted and turned his life upside down and how he has fought back. This book also gives information and signposts sufferers to outside resources enabling them to seek further support. I wish him well in raising fibromyalgia awareness and with this wonderful book.

Michelle Cardno Llb (Hons)
Fightback4Justice-Founder

Contents

Introduction

This book explores my true journey from the very beginning. Having an invisible illness can be very tormenting to your well-being and those around you. You cannot see fibromyalgia and the destruction it causes to oneself.

Having fibromyalgia has left me losing friends, relationships, my job and social life. It has however, taught me that having a little understanding of this condition, has gone a long way to overcoming obstacles that fibromyalgia brings, and has gone a long way to having a better attitude towards myself.

We cannot put our lives on hold and wait for that miracle cure! With a little positive attitude anything and everything is possible to improve our quality of life.

Taking medication helps, but does not always hold the answers. By taking a step by step attitude we can all learn new ways of helping ourselves by coping just that little bit better.

Many fibromyalgia sufferers have their own demons to face. Sometimes it is very hard to even think, or act on looking for ways to be positive as the pain and symptoms, does not give up tormenting us daily. But we have to try and start somewhere.

Having fibromyalgia is a horrific illness, and it is the incurable disease that I have the misfortune of suffering from.

1

Before Fibromyalgia

I left school in 1987, then decided to gain some extra qualifications as I wanted to be a chef. I had always had a fascination in food science. After two years of being on the Youth Training Scheme I was placed into my first ever job. I was ecstatic! Then followed college for further education in home economics, where I gained even more qualifications. From there my cooking was really beginning to take shape.

At this stage, life really was treating me well. I had a career, a job, and my finances were healthy. Best of all I had excellent health, and my future was bright. I had everything going for me. I was enjoying life to the full: late nights out clubbing—which was most weekends, partying with friends and family members, meeting new people.

I travelled abroad, just like any other person. I was filled with an abundance of positive energy that I couldn't get enough of. Nothing seemed to be a problem. There were no obstacles to overcome, no money worries, jobs were easy to obtain—out of one job and into another.

My career was really on the up and up and went from strength to strength. I just loved cooking. It was my life. Everything kept falling into place. Things were perfectly just fine and I was where I wanted to be. Yes! Life was really treating me well.

After various jobs in the catering trade I picked up a lot of catering knowledge, which I will never forget. I had spent the best part of thirteen years being a chef.

As time went by I decided it was time for a career change, as I was still young and wanted to experience other things outside my comfort zone, which I was used to for so long.

In the year 2000, I landed a job as a groundsman for a motorhome company looking after their site grounds. WOW! This was certainly different to what I had become used to. The job was awesome. Working outside in the fresh air all day, what more could I ask for? As all those long days of hours cooped up in a hot sweltering kitchen became a thing of the past, I was again filled with an abundance of positive energy that I couldn't get enough of.

I was so happy. I loved the job. I loved running around, being outside, and listening to the birds singing in the trees, and smelling nature's aromas. With the wind blowing through my hair it was all so relaxing. I loved meeting and talking to different people who visited the site grounds which was a small courtesy part of my job. After only a short-time I picked up more qualifications in ground maintenance. Could life get any better? The money was excellent! I was buying what I wanted when I wanted! Basically, I was living life to the full like I always had done previously.

After five years I became site foreman after a fellow workman retired. I was unstoppable. I knew exactly what I wanted, and how to achieve my goals in order to obtain them; and this was all through working hard—being on time, never late, doing exactly what was expected of me in my job role.

BUT UNBEKNOWN TO ME,

MY LIFE WAS ABOUT

TO TAKE A DRASTIC TURN

FOR THE WORSE.

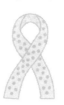

2

When Fibromyalgia Took The First Bite

Predicting the future ... I think we all wished we had the capability to do this. Turning back time is not an option. We can only live with what we know, feel and have experienced.

It was a frosty and seriously cold morning as I cycled to work. I had cycled religiously for the last thirteen years. I covered over two hundred miles a month. I thought I was fit and active. How wrong could I have been!

The years passed by and I wasn't getting any younger! I arrived at work and parked my bike in the designated area. All of a sudden I felt a pain in my left arm. It felt like I had been bitten by something with sharp teeth—these were the only words to express how the pain felt. After a few minutes the intensive pain vanished. This left me wondering. Something wasn't quite right. I had never experienced such severe pain.

As the day went on, what had happened that morning played on my mind. I never complained about things, but this had left me wondering what it was. I had a look at my arm, but there were no scratches or puncture marks! During the day, the intense pain never returned. This, I dismissed as being nothing, and carried on duly completing my duties. However, my subconscious was telling me to get it looked at, but silly me, I did nothing.

A few days passed with no such pain happening again. Until one morning, the pain returned again; the feeling of being bitten. But this time the pain travelled down to my fingertips. Then I realised something was seriously wrong. I was extremely worried, so after work I went to hospital. Whilst waiting to see the doctor, my mind raced, desperately thinking about what could be causing this pain.

After an hour's wait they called, 'Shayne to room five please. Doctor will be with you shortly!' The doctor arrived soon after and asked what the problem was. I explained that I had been getting sharp, stabbing pains down my left arm. After examining my arm he said, 'Shayne, I think you have pulled a muscle!' Phew! What a relief, as I was convinced it was something more ominous. No medication was given. I thanked the doctor and upon leaving was advised to take a generic pain killer, and that this should settle down in a couple of weeks. Off I went, quite satisfied.

After a few weeks the pain was getting worse, and so severe I couldn't take anymore. I finished work and off to the hospital I went. This time I saw a different doctor who ran some tests - these came back normal. I guess the pulled muscle hadn't quite healed. Weeks passed and after another two trips to the hospital I thought, 'Right, the time has come for me to speak up and find out what was going on!'

On my fifth visit to the hospital, I was given some insight as to what might be causing the pain. The doctor mentioned "FIBROMYALGIA" and didn't think it was a pulled muscle after all. My eyes opened wide in shock! I had never heard of fibromyalgia before, and I don't think many people had. I asked the doctor numerous questions, but I was referred to my GP with the explanation, 'We are only trained in accident and emergency!'

I made an online appointment to see my GP.
The morning of my appointment arrived and I was anxious to find out what fibromyalgia was. I could have looked on the internet of course, but this could only confuse matters and make my anxiety worse.

I explained to my GP what had been happening and my numerous visits to the hospital; stating the last doctor I saw said it might be fibromyalgia. My GP ran some blood tests, checked my heart, lungs and breathing—which were fine, and said, 'Let's get the results of the bloods back and take it from there, and if you have any more problems to come back.' A few days passed and the blood tests came back, normal. The GP dismissed me with the words, 'See how you go.'
During the next few months the pain exacerbated. I felt sick and now other problems appeared:

- Fatigued all the time
- Dizziness

- Aching
- Feeling stiff
- Frequent headaches/migraines
- Pains in the hands
- Going hot then cold
- Literally dripping with sweat
- Stomach pains
- Sore gums
- Pain in the jaw
- Difficulty concentrating
- Neck pain
- Walking became difficult
- Loss of hand grip
- Muscle spasms
- Numbness in fingers
- Acid reflux
- Involuntary falling over

Sleep was almost impossible. The stress of all this began to take hold. It was taking a toll on my health. This had happened in the space of three months from experiencing the first bite of pain!

WHEN YOU HURT SO BADLY,

YOU STRUGGLE TO EVEN

BREATHE,

MOVE, OR CRY

3

My First Visit To The Rheumatologist

One Tuesday morning I was woken by the letter box being slammed hard. I felt half dazed and dizzy as I hadn't had much sleep. It was at that moment I realised that sleep deprivation was in full force and the fatigue was beginning to show. I thought, 'Oh, it must be the postman!', and laid in bed for a while longer until I was more alert and gradually came to my senses.

These days it was becoming increasingly hard to wake up properly. In the past, this was never a problem; as soon as I woke up, I was alert and ready to face whatever the day had in store for me.

I managed to crawl out of bed, tip toed down stairs as it was early, and I didn't want to wake the rest of my family up. I had to lean heavily on the banisters—my balance was so out of control. When I eventually got to the bottom step, I noticed a large pile of mail had been delivered. At this moment, I was trying my hardest to be alert. I was so tired, my eyes were barely open, and my focus was at a minimum. As I bent down to pick up the mail I felt extremely dizzy. This had became a regular occurrence. I looked through the mail and noticed one for me. I began to open the letter and saw that a local medical centre was mentioned. Curious as to what this was, I sat down and started to read. It appeared my doctor had made me an appointment at my local medical centre. I thought, 'Oh, wow! My doctor had actually taken notice and wanted further investigations!' The appointment was in a few days' time.

The day arrived and my Dad and myself got in the car, as he was taking me there. On arrival, I checked in at reception and waited. After a few minutes my name was called. I did not know what to expect as I was feeling very anxious. The rheumatologist explained that my own doctor was concerned about my health and that is why I was there. After a few general health questions he explained that he was going to examine various parts of my anatomy. The examination started. He pressed various parts of my body. My response was, 'Oh, God that hurt!' He carried on and my responses were, 'Ouch! That hurt!'

We sat down after the examination and I waited for what came next. He said, 'Shayne, you have all the symptoms of what can only be described as fibromyalgia.' On the way home I thought, 'At least I had a diagnosis now.'

A few days later the patient copy of the rheumatologist's report came. His findings were:

- Multiple trigger points
- Exertional fatigue
- Associated nail dystrophy
- ANA, rheumatoid and thyroid functions test - negative

As I was reading this report I saw that the rheumatologist had referred me to the Fibromyalgia Educational Programme, which was as held at my local hospital. This would be conducted with two senior physiotherapists trained in rheumatology. This would turn out to be very beneficial.

YOU CAN'T ALWAYS

SEE THE PAIN

SOMEONE FEELS

4

What I Know About Fibromyalgia

Around 1 in 50 people develop fibromyalgia at some point in their life.

Fibromyalgia: also known as Fibromyalgia Syndrome (FMS). This condition is not classed as a disease, but rather a neurological condition where inappropriate nerve signals produced in the brain cause symptoms in the body.

Fibromyalgia is a debilitating chronic condition that causes widespread muscle pain. It can affect every part of the body! The pain mainly occurs in the tendons, and ligaments. As well as other symptoms and associated symptoms, it can lead the sufferer to complete isolation.

Fibromyalgia is a long term condition where the symptoms can be treated, but, they never go away completely. This means the sufferer can experience a long agonising pain up to five times the level of non-sufferers. This in turn can, and does lead to severe stress, anxiety and depression.

Diagnosing fibromyalgia can be very difficult as there is no specific test and the symptoms can vary significantly from person to person. A diagnosis is made by exclusion of other conditions with similar symptoms to fibromyalgia, and it can therefore take a long time to reach a point of a diagnosis. A diagnosis is usually made by medical history and a trigger point test on certain points of the body. Also blood tests, a trigger point test, X-rays and other scans maybe performed to rule out other conditions before a diagnosis is actually made. Sometimes it can take years of suffering to get a diagnosis of fibromyalgia.

In the past, fibromyalgia has been known by different names:

- Fibromyositis
- Fibrositis
- Muscular Rheumatism
- Musculoskeletal Pain Syndrome

Fibromyalgia has been said not to cause any harm to other organs of the body. But many sufferers have disputed this. It is said that it does not affect your life span.

1 in 25 people develop fibromyalgia (patient.info/health/fibromyalgia-leaflet)

It's not what you look at that really matters, it's what you see.
Fibromyalgia is an invisible illness YOU CANNOT SEE.
What you see on the outside isn't what's happening on the inside?
WE LOOK NORMAL.
Just because you can't see something doesn't mean it's not there.

5

The Symptoms Of Fibromyalgia

Fibromyalgia can cause your body to ache all over. In extreme conditions this can appear as flu-like symptoms. Other symptoms are crippling fatigue and agonising pain, especially in tender parts of the body known as "trigger points". The pain is extremely agonising. This illness can also cause sleep deprivation, aching and severe pain around the muscle joints, which include the neck, shoulders, back and hips.

Other symptoms may include:

- Widespread muscle pain
- Headaches/migraine
- Irritable Bowel Syndrome (IBS)
- Forgetfulness or poor quality of concentration (Fibro Fog)
- Numbness in hands and feet
- Poor circulation
- Restless Leg Syndrome (medical term - Willis-Ekbom disease)
- Dry mouth
- Stiffness and dizziness

- Frequent urination
- Crying for no apparent reason
- Sweating
- Involuntary muscle twitching
- Teeth grinding (bruxism)
- Runny nose
- Tinnitus
- Constant itching
- Stress and anxiety
- Depression
- Chronic Fatigue Syndrome (CFS)
- Dry eye syndrome

The actual cause of fibromyalgia has always been an unknown mystery due to the complexities of this condition, but there are a number of potential theories that are presented at this time. Research has shown there maybe multiple factors involved in the onset of this condition. Other possible causes are:

- Viral infection
- Physical injury
- Lack of exercise
- Altered pain perception
- Defective gene
- Lack of growth hormone

Unfortunately, at this time there is no cure, but researchers and scientists are working really hard to find new treatments and medication with fewer side effects, with the aim to ease the symptoms and to improve our quality of life.

THERE ARE OVER

200 FIBROMYALGIA

ASSOCIATED SYMPTOMS

18 Tender Points
(also known as *The Trigger Points*)

Right base of skull
Neck & shoulder right
Right upper inner shoulder

Left base of skull
Neck & shoulder left
Left upper inner shoulder

Right outer upper buttock
Right hip bone

Left outer upper buttock
Left hip bone

Back of Body

Lower right neck in front
Lower left neck in front
Edge left of upper chest

Edge right of upper chest

Below right bone side at elbow

Below right bone side at elbow

Just above knee on inside

Just above knee on inside

Rheumatology guidelines suggest that people with fibromyalgia have pain in at least 11 of these tender points when a doctor applies a certain amount of pressure.

Front of Body

6

"OH–NO!"
Not Irritable Bowel Syndrome (IBS)

Not only was I fighting against the horrifying fibromyalgia—there was something else! I was having problems with my digestive system! Most mornings I would wake up with excruciating abdominal pain, severe cramps and bloating. Every time I had something to eat - within minutes - I had to go and empty my bowels! So, guess what? Once again, back to the doctors. Trips to the doctor were becoming a regular part of my life.

An examination, more blood tests and stool tests. The marks were high from the stool test and certainly indicated Irritable Bowel Syndrome. By this time I was feeling really down. How much more could one person take? Even more medication was prescribed and off I went with tears in my eyes. I began the slow walk home trying to absorb even more problems. I wondered why this was happening to me.

After arriving home I decided to research what Irritable Bowel Syndrome (IBS) was, and what could be done other than taking medication. Amongst numerous searches I discovered that

Irritable Bowel Syndrome can be related to having fibromyalgia. They often happen together, but how they are related is still not yet completely understood. With both conditions, you have more brain activity in the parts that process pain. Your sense of pain can be enhanced. Having these two disorders together, your nervous system becomes overly sensitive or hyperactive.

The more you know about and understand Irritable Bowel Syndrome, the better you can start to get relief. The good news is that (IBS) can be managed. As time goes on it does become easier to identify the triggers, and so many people find that their symptoms can become less severe over time.

There are three types of Irritable Bowel Syndrome:

- Irritable Bowel Syndrome (C) Constipation (IBS-C)
- Irritable Bowel Syndrome (D) Diarrhoea (IBS-D)
- Irritable Bowel Syndrome (M) Mixed constipation and diarrhoea (IBS-M)

WHEN TOILET PAPER

BECOMES YOUR BEST FRIEND

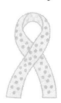

7

Why Me?

I often sat and wondered, 'What had I done in my earlier life that was so drastically wrong that I ended up with this misery and suffering?' I spent days thinking about the time when I was fit and active. Had I missed something that I never picked up early enough in life?

My thoughts were:

- Did my days of partying and drinking cause this?
- Did smoking cause this?
- Was my diet at fault?
- Had my working life of early mornings and late nights cause this?
- Was I not as fit and active that I thought I was?
- Did medication cause this?
- Did working hard cause this?
- Is it genetic?
- Did my ancestors have it?
- Did I have a mental trauma?

So many thoughts were going through my mind trying to find a link. I had spent years researching and studying my medical and life history. There appeared to be a connection for me having fibromyalgia, and that turned out to possibly be STRESS.

Stress is a silent killer in the body which can affect everyone. If you are not showing any signs or symptoms it can still be working its magical devastation on the inside. One day it could just erupt like it did to me. The worst thing is, I never saw it coming!

My case is just one possible cause of fibromyalgia. Remember, fibromyalgia can hit men, women and children—yes, children. It hits hard. If you are not sure, but you begin to show any signs of fibromyalgia, get it checked as this can often mimic signs of other illnesses.

WHY DO THINGS ALWAYS

HAPPEN TO ME?

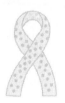

HOW ARE YOU?

HURTING. TIRED. SCARED. CONFUSED.
LONELY. CRUSHED. DEPRESSED. EMPTY.
HELPLESS. FRAGILE. WEAK. HOPELESS.
MISERABLE. DAZED. FRUSTRATED. ANGRY.
HEARTBROKEN. TORMENTED. WOUNDED.
COMFORTLESS. CAST OUT. LOUSEY. IN DESPAIR.
FOGGY BRAIN. OFF BALANCE.
SICK. TIRED OF BEING SICK.

AND PEOPLE THINK WE MAKE THIS UP.
TRY LIVING WITH FIBROMYALGIA

8

Time For Medication

Over the next and coming months I travelled back and forth to the doctors. Time progressed and I was trying to ingest eleven different types of medication. These ranged from:

- Neuropathic pain killers
- Non –benzodiazepine hypnotic agent drugs
- Non-steroidal anti-inflammatory drugs
- Selective serotonin reuptake inhibitors
- Colecalciferol (Vitamin D3 supplements)
- Proton pump inhibitors
- Intestinal bladder spasm drugs

I could not believe that such an illness could cause such devastation to me and lead to taking so many medications just to try and manage the condition. I felt like a walking pill bottle. Never in my wildest dreams could I have imagined I would end up being so sick and debilitated and to be taking so many drugs to fix a problem, but couldn't. I was horrified to the worst degree and my health was spiralling out of control.

I FELT LIKE

A WALKING PHARMACY

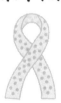

9

My First Hand Experience With Side-Effects

We all know that medication can cause side effects, but, not everybody experiences them. With me, it was a totally different story. I list mine below:

- Detached from reality
- Vivid nightmares
- Abnormal night sweats
- Blurred vision
- Tremors
- Aggression
- Weight gain
- Loss of taste
- Low mood
- Irritable, fidgety
- Loss of appetite
- Nausea
- Constant dry mouth
- Drowsiness
- Confusion
- Constipation

- Stomach ache
- Constant itching

Once the medication had been changed a majority of the side-effects disappeared. They didn't return or cause any long time or lasting side effects.

If you feel that one or another medication gives you nasty side effects, there will be more you can try that may suit you with less side effects. This is trial and error. What suits one doesn't suit everybody.

THE SIDE-EFFECTS

ARE SOMETIMES

WORSE THAN THE PAIN

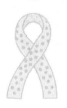

10

Visits To The Neurologist

I was experiencing a vast amount of problems plus new symptoms. I was dealing with them but they didn't seem to be improving. My doctor took the decision to refer me to a neurologist for further investigation.

I had shooting pains across my face, electric shock type sensations in my mouth and across the jaws, numbness in my right hand, involuntary jerking of my arms and legs. Fatigue hadn't improved, and my feet and hands were swelling with a burning sensation. I had constant body aches and balance problems.

As a precaution these tests were undertaken:

- EEG - Electroencephalogram
- MRI - Magnetic Resonance Imaging
- Blood tests which revealed low level vitamin D

At this part of my journey, I really felt like a human guinea pig. The majority of these tests were coming back normal. There was still no indication why I was experiencing so many problems, apart from the words, "it's fibromyalgia". I'm in contact with my neurologist on a regular basis to help try and relieve my symptoms.

YOU CAN'T ALWAYS

SEE THE PAIN

SOMEONE FEELS

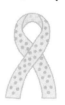

11

Fibromyalgia Training Programme

A letter arrived giving me the date of my first visit to the physiotherapists for the Fibromyalgia Educational Programme. This would be held at my local hospital where, I hoped to learn more about this tormenting and destructive illness.

The course lasted eight weeks and this is what I learnt:

- Fibromyalgia exercises
- Coping
- Pain management
- Stress management:
- Diaphragmatic breathing
- Sleep deprivation
- Importance of posture
- Communication and lifestyle
- Healthy eating
- How to manage symptoms
- Pacing
- Support groups

I learnt important information that would be invaluable in the ensuing weeks. I recall there were about ten others in the group. Ages varied; some with the same problem as me. Some had walking aids, some could hardly walk, some were in pain and crying mainly because they were so overwhelmed. There were also some struggling to get to grips with the exercises; it was just too much for them. As an onlooker I knew exactly what they were feeling.

The course taught me that not everyone with fibromyalgia suffered in the same way. Each week on this programme I found that some people never turned up. I could only think they were suffering and couldn't make it.

There were weeks when aches and pains were awful, but I told myself, 'Come on, Shayne, you can do it!' Each lesson lasted two hours. Even within this period I felt pain, exhaustion, irritability and fidgety. There were times when my brain didn't seem capable of absorbing information properly anymore. This frustrated me. But, each time I carried on regardless.

The physiotherapists running the programme were very knowledgeable and knew exactly what we were going through. They had an exceptional understanding of our problems and helped where they could.

I was really fed up when the programme finished as I wouldn't see the group of people again. We all took each other's contact numbers when we parted, but I lost that piece of paper with the numbers on. These people got to know me, and me them. They became my friends, even for such a small period of time. This meant a lot, because they knew first-hand what I was going through. The sad part was, I never did find that piece of paper and couldn't meet them again, and because my mobile phone was upgraded shortly after and my number had changed, they couldn't contact me either.

The time had come for me to put this new found knowledge into action. Over the next few months I tried everything. Some things worked and some didn't. I was so desperate to manage this illness and live a normal life, but it wasn't going to happen! This illness wasn't going anywhere. The more I tried, the worse I was. It was three steps forward and two steps back. This went on for months and I just couldn't get complete relief. It was soul destroying and making me mentally and physically ill.

I had to do something! My initial thoughts were the internet. Surely there had to be other things I could try. After all, this illness had been around since the 1800s. There had to be more about it out there, something to be discovered and tried other than what I had been told.

I made it my mission to trawl the internet looking for answers! I spent two years looking every day but there was nothing there. Of course, fibromyalgia was mentioned on hundreds of websites. Where were the answers I desperately wanted to see? I wanted relief; the torment of this illness was becoming unbearable! I couldn't cope with the pain, the aches, and everything that fibromyalgia threw at me on a daily basis. I began to think, I'm doomed for destruction, but all the time...

MY SUBCONSCIOUS

WAS TELLING ME

TO KEEP TRYING

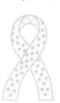

12

My Exercise Programme

Briefly, this is what I was trying to achieve at home:

- Bring each knee to chest, one after the other
- Walk hands up against the wall
- Circulating arms upwards
- Sit and stand up
- Lift a hand weight from side to side whilst sitting
- Walking up and down the bedroom
- Throw and catch a ball against the wall
- Swing legs backwards and forwards and alternate
- Standing on tiptoes
- Push ups against the wall
- Facial arthromyalgia mouth exercises (added at a later date)

After leaving the Fibromyalgia Therapy Programme I tried to do some of the above exercises daily. I tried as often and when I could, but most days this wasn't possible as the fatigue and pain were too much to handle. I did try and work through the best I could. I was taught that exercising can decrease the pain. Some days I was just so stiff, I could hardly move to get out of bed let alone do anything else; exercises were the last thing on my mind.

I noticed a few days later that after managing to do a few of these exercises, the aches and pains weren't too bad. However, the next day did I suffer! The aches and pains seemed to be at an all-time high, and I couldn't understand why, then I remembered "pacing".

THREE STEPS FORWARD

TWO STEPS BACK

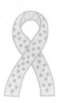

13

Pacing Myself

As I remembered, pacing is all about spreading tasks evenly rather that doing everything in one go. I had to limit myself and take breaks in between what I was doing. Even this was difficult. I needed a routine but, I couldn't get into one. My symptoms were acting up all the time and it was extremely hard to find a routine that worked around me, my aches and pains.

Fatigue was preventing me from doing almost anything. I just seemed to lie on my bed because I felt so poorly! With the constant fatigue along with the aches and pains I could hardly move. I had poor balance and lying prone on my bed seemed to be part of my daily routine. What else could I do?

The days passed and it got to the stage where I couldn't manage to do anything, and I thought that I would do it tomorrow; but as we all know, tomorrow never comes.

It got to the stage when I couldn't manage to do much at all. It came to the point where I wasn't getting dressed until mid-morning. Getting dressed was becoming a task in itself, so I just lied on my bed watching TV or trawled the internet on my phone. This is how this illness was affecting me. All the time I was in pain, aching and fatigued. For whatever reason, I was questioning my medication, was I on the right ones?

This illness wasn't affecting my appearance to say there was something wrong with me, though. Even this was something I couldn't understand. Normally when you are ill, your appearance alters. With fibromyalgia it doesn't work that way, and this can be very misleading to a lot a people. We look a picture of health.

I DON'T HAVE TO GO FAST,

I JUST HAVE TO REST IN BETWEEN

14

When I Turned To Social Media

I already had two accounts on the social media networks, but I never bothered using them. All I could see were people bitching about each other, people being scammed for money. At this particular time I thought, 'No! This isn't for me.'

After a long time deliberating about this, I decided to go back to social media. I already knew there were sites for different things. I never gave it another thought to look any further to see if there were sites for fibromyalgia. Why should I? I hadn't been diagnosed with it yet!

I typed in fibromyalgia and sat back and waited.

I was shocked. There were numerous sites. I didn't count them; I would have been there all day. I did discover however, that the majority of these sites had between 6000 - 15000 members. I couldn't believe what I was seeing. There were so many people suffering from this illness.

I quickly started looking through the sites, reading a few group profile headings. I noticed that some of them stated, "we are a fibromyalgia support group and here to support anyone who has this debilitating condition". In an instant I asked to join. By the time I had finished I had joined over eighty groups; I was so desperate for information.

After a few weeks had passed of looking at these groups, I noticed that they were full of women. I thought to myself, 'Where are all the men? Surely I can't be the only man with fibromyalgia!'

I found a few men had joined after me, but weren't saying much. I also found out that fibromyalgia was classed as a "woman's illness". Men found it an embarrassment to be associated with this. Yes, I thought, I can understand this—why would a man want a woman's illness without sounding condescending?

In the group I came across a lady who was talking about men with fibromyalgia, and according to her, 1 in 7 men are estimated to have fibromyalgia. I also learnt that over 2.7 million people in Great Britain suffer with fibromyalgia (fibromyalgiasyndrome. com.uk, 2013), and this number is growing larger every day. I was really gobsmacked! Further reading showed that 75 - 90% of women were affected (fibromyalgiasyndrome.com.uk, 2013). It is much more common in women!

After a period of time I decided to set up my own support group. I just couldn't be bothered with flitting from group and group. My group was growing at a fast pace; more members joining every day and they come from all over the world. The idea of this support group was to help and empower fibromyalgia sufferers to talk to other people. Some are housebound and don't get to speak to other people very often. I have met lots of friends since starting this group. They are all such genuine people.

Some of us have met up and shared stories. Finally I was with people who understood me and what I was going through. It really made a difference and my self-esteem returned to an all-time high. I even started dating again; something I hadn't done for years. My self-confidence was gradually coming back.

15

When Sleeping Became A Nightmare

Sleeping was beginning to become a major problem. I was constantly struggling with fatigue and could not get a restful night's sleep. The pain and the body aches were becoming a nightmare and they were preventing me from sleeping. When I finally got to sleep, my arms and legs would jerk—this was so uncomfortable. I was already dealing with so much and all I wanted to do was sleep. I was exhausted. I felt like a walking zombie.

On average I was getting 2-3 hours of disturbed sleep. The mornings were awful. I felt so ill that I had to go back to the doctor— even more medication—but only for a week. This medication was addictive and he did not want me becoming an addict as I was already dealing with so much in my life.

I took my first tablet, and no kidding, within twenty minutes my eyes were closing. Wow! This stuff was really potent. It literally knocked me out! That night I slept like a log. I slept like I hadn't done for years. Over the course of a week I was sleeping, but, when the medication stopped I was back to square one! The next day I phoned the doctor for some more, but he wouldn't give me anymore, stating they were addictive and sent me a leaflet on how to get a better sleep.

This leaflet explained why people with fibromyalgia had disturbed sleep and woke up feeling unrefreshed. Taking sleeping tablets wasn't the answer; they didn't work for long and left you feeling tired and irritable the next day. They also tend to lose their effect quite quickly, hence the reason why they tend to be addictive. They should only be used for short periods - less than two weeks.

Reading through the leaflet, it mentioned that a percentage of people who suffer from severe tiredness could be a contributory factor of Myalgia Encephalomyelitis (ME) or Chronic Fatigue Syndrome (CFS). As time went on, I found out that ME or CFS is a related condition that can be present in people with fibromyalgia. I was now on a mission to find out all I could about these conditions and what could be done.

16

When Working Was A "NO-NO"

Halfway through my journey, I was still struggling to come to terms with fibromyalgia and its devastation on my health. I was still working, and, I was now diagnosed with Meniere's disease, which is also known as Endolymphatic Hydrops; a rare disease of unknown cause. This disease affects the labyrinth of the inner ear and can cause hearing loss to deafness, attacks of vertigo and tinnitus.

As I carried on researching I came across some information that said fibromyalgia sufferers have a 75% chance of developing Meniere's disease. Great I thought. What else is round the corner? The flood gates were now really wide open for the potential attacks of other conditions to be encountered. Work started to be virtually impossible dealing with these two illnesses. I thought enough was enough! The days of my working life were almost over. I didn't know what to do!

I met with Human Resources Management and it was mutually agreed that, it was time for me to finish work. This was such a sad time for me, as I loved my job, but, what else could I do?

My health was really suffering because of these illnesses. I finished work and said goodbye to my work mates. They wished me luck for the future and hoped I'd get well. The time had come for me to sign on as sick, but this was only going to last a year!

Now the nightmare began! Where was I going to get 'money' from, and how would I survive? I still had bills to pay, and they weren't going to go away! All I knew about money was - you worked to get money. What was I going to do? I knew nothing about "state benefits", or how to claim them? I had always worked. Where did I go? What did I do? Nobody had ever told me! Phone call after phone call—it was time to claim social security.

Stress was really beginning to affect me. I had no money coming in, and what money I did have was what I had from work. That money wasn't going to last forever. At this point my parents helped support me the best they could.

The days and weeks passed and the bills were piling up and I just couldn't pay them! I had to start selling things I'd worked hard for. At this point, the stress was hitting me really hard; I didn't need this worry.

At last the forms arrived to claim social assistance. The forms I had to fill out were psychologically stressful to the maximum. My mind just couldn't function as it was. Hours passed and I had finally filled the forms and posted them back.

It wasn't going to stop there though, oh no! A few weeks passed when news arrived in the post! An appointment had been made for me to go and see the Department for Works and Pensions (DWP) for a medical. I was thinking, who are these people? I had never heard of them before!

When the day of my appointment arrived, I had never felt so insulted or disbelieved in all my life about how my illness was having such an impact on my health. I knew these people had a job to do, but, where was the courtesy! They asked question after question. I couldn't believe the amount they were asking! All I wanted to do was to get help. I was told finally, I could get Employment and Support Allowance. I was placed into the work related group. After a year, I had to go back and see them again. I had a medical to justify whether I was fit for work. After the medical, they found me fit for work! My mouth dropped in disbelief. How had they come to this conclusion? I was seriously suffering. I had already finished work because I could no longer fulfil my duties. The increased stress of this process really made me ill and my fibromyalgia symptoms were increasing and I just wasn't coping at all.

Another letter arrived, but this time it was to see a Work Programme Advisor. One thing led to another, and well over a year had passed going backwards and forwards. I now appealed to DWP and was finally placed into the support group for ESA. Phew! It only took three years of chronic ill health to be believed.

Now that some of the pressure was off, my stress levels was now manageable. However, on the other hand, I was still finding it hard to deal with my illness ...

I`M NOT LAZY

- I`M SICK

FIBROMYALGIA

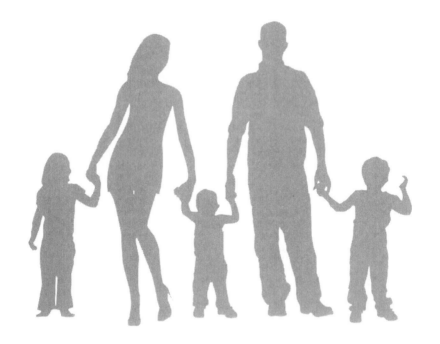

CAN AFFECT
MEN, WOMEN
AND CHILDREN

17

Let's Look At PIP
(Personal Independence Payment)

Guide to Personal Independence Payment:

Personal Independence Payment is a UK Government benefit for those who are aged between 16 and 64. It is to help with the costs of your disability.

PIP is not awarded on the disability you have, but, on the effects of your day to day activities.

- You must meet a certain criteria's of PIP
- You can claim PIP if you are working or not
- The benefit is non means tested and is not taxable

For those who are having a future PIP assessment, or those who are thinking of applying:

- Make sure you have all your medical notes to hand
- What medication you take - this should be a list of present

and past medications. This will indicate you are under your doctor for your illness or illnesses.

It is worth noting what professionals you have seen:

- Physiotherapist
- Rheumatologist
- Counselling
- Mental Health Team
- Pain Management etc. etc.

What treatment have they advised for you? Maybe you have letters to confirm you have seen them. Show them those letters. Also, get copies of your patient notes from the professionals you have seen.

When you have an assessment, these assessors do not know you, they can only assess you on the information you give them for the outcome of the decision. Also, remember it is not the assessor who makes the final decision. You must tell them everything. Some of these assessors do not have full medical training in fibromyalgia.

- You need to look as you would on a typical day
- Don't hide your pain, let them see your pain
- If you are fidgety, then fidget
- If you can't make eye contact, then don't
- Cry if you need to
- If you feel nervous, be nervous
- Don't cover anything up!

Remember, we are good at covering things up, DON'T.
Let the assessor see the real you. Tell them how you feel and struggle every day.

They will ask you lots of questions on how your illness/illnesses affects you. This is your chance to tell them how you feel. Don't miss anything out—the slightest thing will make every difference.

Example:

- If your partner or family help you, then tell them.
Maybe your husband/partner/wife/family member helps you wash as you can't lift your arms because of pain and stiffness.

- Maybe you need assistance to go to the toilet, as you need to hold on to them because of balance problems. If your illness affects you this way, you find it hard getting off the toilet.

- Maybe you can't cook for yourself as you can't stand long enough because of pain, dizziness and you lose concentration. Maybe you have burnt yourself previously.

- Maybe you find it difficult to get out of the house, because you can't walk very far because you have to stop and get your breath and the pain cripples you.

- Maybe you suffer with anxiety and depression and this stops you leaving the house.

• Tell them how fibromyalgia affects your movement and co-ordination.

• Maybe you struggle to get out of bed, or spend days in bed.

• Maybe you find yourself sleeping all the time, or you don't sleep for days.

Every word will count. Never lie or bend the truth. Be honest and have creditable evidence to back up everything you mentioned about how your illness/illnesses affect you in detail.

NOTE: *This guide does not cover all circumstances. For more details, look on the UK Government website.*

Michelle Cardno Llb (Hons) is an expert in her field of welfare benefits. This lady and her team will put you on the right track if you need further assistance. Contact her on the useful addresses page.

NOTHING GOOD EVER COMES

FROM BEING DISHONEST

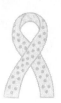

18

Let's Talk "Fibro Fog"

Fibro fog is also known as brain fog. These words are used when you have cognitive difficulties. This is a feeling of being in a daze—you feel like your brain is working backwards. This can come as a shock if you have not experienced it before. This was another symptom I felt up against.

One time I left the gas on under the grill section of the cooker. I walked away not realising I had left it on—until the fire alarm went off. The cooker was hot and smoking, and took a long time to clear. It almost left me in tears. This fog can leave you very disorientated and severely confused. In my mind I thought I had turned the gas off. This was happening regularly with different things. Everything I did from now I checked 2-3 times. My brain just could not comprehend what I was doing.

Reading was difficult. It felt like my eyes were skipping lines. My mind just couldn't take in information or process it properly. The simplest of words I couldn't read or spell. I was forgetting friend's names, but yet, I always used to speak to them. Most days the words, 'What's your name?' crossed my mind! I didn't dare say to them in case they thought I had lost the plot! I felt that my jaw wasn't connected to my brain. My quality of speech was all muddled up. It made sense to me, but not to the people who were listening to me.

One day I was making a drink and waited for the kettle to boil. I must have stood in a daze, waiting ages but it never boiled. I thought the fuse must have blown. I checked the fuse in another plug and it worked. It took me ages to actually figure out why the kettle didn't work! Yes, you guessed right, I hadn't turned the kettle on.

There seems to be a correlation with fibromyalgia and fibro fog. Fibro fog can go from mild to the extreme. Not everyone will experience the cognitive difficulties. It is said that stress, poor sleep and medication can also be a contributory factor.

Fibro fog can manifest itself in different ways in different people. Some of the most common symptoms I've experienced are:

- Short term memory loss
- Misplacing objects
- Becoming easily distracted
- Not being able to put a sentence together
- Inability to remember new information
- Not remembering names
- Disorientation (get lost easily)
- Poor ability to give directions

- Right-left confusion
- Difficulty understanding what you've read
- Difficulty calculating simple maths sums
- Difficulty spelling simple words

NOT EVERY

FIBROMYALGIA SUFFERER

WILL EXPERIENCE

THESE SYMPTOMS

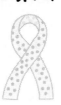

19

Open Wide Please

Over time I was noticing that the pain was moving. Not only was it affecting my arms, legs, hands, back, feet and neck, the pain was working its way to my face. I initially thought I had tooth ache. I had never experienced pain like it in my face. The pain was affecting every inch of my body. A trip to the dentist was in order.

After the dentist completed her examination she said, 'Shayne, your teeth are fine. I'm sorry to say you have all the symptoms of Temporomandibular Joint Dysfunction (TMJD).' She also said that I should see a maxillofacial surgeon for a more in-depth investigation. I had clicking both sides of my jaw. It was painful to palpate masseter muscles, and also painful to palpate with limited opening. The dentist suggested that I use non-steroid anti-inflammatory cream on the joints of the jaw. I had to use this until I saw the surgeon.

The day arrived and after telling the surgeon what the dentist had said, and explaining how I was feeling in my face, my face examination began. 'Open wide please ... now I'm going to insert my thumbs right up the jaw and gently push both sides of your masseter muscles.' I let out on almighty scream. Sweat literally poured from my face. The pain was so severe I almost fainted. I was in sheer agony.

The surgeon said it wasn't TMJD, but a form of TMJD, which shows all the signs and same symptoms; it is known as Facial Arthromyalgia! The same family, but with a different disorder. He explained that this is related to fibromyalgia and is also caused by stress. I was told that I had to seriously reduce my stress levels and calm down. I explained to him, as I had to other professionals, that I was suffering with so much going on inside me and it was hard to reduce. He gave me four steps in managing jaw pain (explained below) and to carry on using the cream on the jaws. This might help other sufferers with the same problem and it also works with TMJD.

• Rest yourself and your jaw
• Exercise regularly
• Eat soft food - avoid hard foods like nuts, crusty bread or anything that takes a lot of chewing
• Chew on your back teeth not the front ones
• Eat small bites at a time
• Sleep on your side
• Avoid joint or muscle damage by not doing contact sports (wear a mouth guard if you play contact sports)
• Chew gum
• Stop habits such as - biting finger nails, pens, pencils

or lips
- Book long dental appointments
- Play a wind instrument
- Reduce muscle pain with analgesics and by applying cold packs for 10 minutes every 3 hours for 72 hours after injury, hot packs for 20 minutes every 3 hours to injured joints/muscles

NOW to re-educate the jaw opening:

- Open your mouth with a hinged movement
- Exercise your jaw twice daily, opening 5 times in front of a mirror ensuring the jaw opens vertically downwards without deviating side-wards.

Exercise your jaw 3 times daily timed for 5 minutes:

- Close your mouth on the back teeth
- Put the tip of your tongue on the palate behind your front teeth
- Move the tongue back across the palate as far as it will go
- Keep the tongue in this position with the teeth closed for 10 seconds
- Open your mouth slowly until the tongue starts to leave the palate - keep in that position for 10 seconds
- Close your mouth
- Repeat over 5 minutes

After several attempts the pain started to decrease. This was now added to my daily regime!

WHEN YOU`RE IN PAIN,

IT'S SAD WHEN YOU CAN SAY,

'IT'S A PART OF MY LIFE NOW'

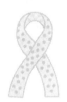

20

Finally Things Started To Turn Around

We know fibromyalgia is a life-long crippling condition and it isn't going to go anywhere fast, but something had to be done. I wasn't going to sit and suffer any longer. Something had to change. I had spent years suffering.

It was back to the beginning. So, I searched and searched through all I'd been taught. Now I had to find solutions. Surely it was here and I was determined. I took the approach of thinking that if I was going to get better, it would be based on my decisions and experiences. Doctors could only do so much, because, after all I was the one living with the condition!

The first steps I took were looking through papers, and I started to absorb what was in front of me. This was in more detail, and word for word. I then put into order what I could realistically do and try to achieve.

This is what I did:

- Understand the condition and symptoms in more depth.
- Pacing from the beginning
- Goal setting
- Graded exercise
- Understanding sleep patterns
- Relaxation techniques
- Deep breathing techniques

In the beginning it was hard to achieve, just like before. This time I was determined not to give up. I had the answers for some relief in front of me. The problem was I just didn't know how to use them.

Over the next couple of weeks, I was finally beginning to see some results. I tried to keep my mind focused all of the time I was doing a task. At the same time, I was, of course battling between symptoms from one place in body to the next.

Sleep had begun to be more regular than 2-3 hours a night, and sleeping through the day wore off. Once I had learnt to do things, relaxation started to become beneficial and exercise increased daily. I began to gather more information from books, specialists, internet journals and also talking to and liaising with people who had this condition.

I was now starting to feel slightly better about myself and stress; well, that was down to being minimal. Aches started to decrease. I started taking vitamins with my meals and drinking more water was introduced into my diet: lack of water is one main trigger of daytime fatigue. Drinking 8-10 glasses of water a day has been shown to ease back and joint pain for up to 80% of sufferers. So, for now, things were finally improving.

21

How To Deal With Fibromyalgia

Coping with fibromyalgia is accepting the fact that the problem is a devastatingly chronic condition. I have learned ways in which to minimise the pain, symptoms and finding the good things I could do. The reality is, the symptoms will never go away completely. We need to learn as much as we can, and put it into practice.

You will find ways of coping better. It took me a while. If you don't find ways to cope better, you will lose your self-confidence. This means that you could end up as an ill, frustrated person. Never think that just because you have fibromyalgia it is the end—IT IS NOT. I learned that I can be strong, even though I have my own limitations. I can still put things into practice, little by little.

When living with fibromyalgia, it is so easy to lose hope and give up. It is easy to breakdown under the pressure that seems to be against us. The truth is, there is always HOPE.

Please remember that you can always do more to improve your

health. You can always see another doctor or specialist. You can seek more treatment, the list just goes on. No matter how bad your symptoms are, you can always try to do something different.

Never give up on looking for HELP. There is so much out there to be learnt and discussed about fibromyalgia. Whatever you can do to help yourselves, will help towards improving your quality of life, and hopefully you will find peace.

The thing about fibromyalgia is that it does not come with an "instruction manual". There are no guarantees and nobody said it was going to be easy.

THERE IS ALWAYS

MORE TO LEARN

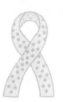

22

Talking With Your Partner

Talk constructively to your partner/family members and carers to discuss your condition, and make decisions that will be workable, beneficial and manageable for all. Be very clear on what you want and the way forward.

When one of you becomes ill with fibromyalgia, it will be life changing. It will be time to compromise with each other and maximise your efforts. You need to be completely honest with each other.

Don't find yourself in a position you will regret because of poor communication. I've seen a lot of couples end their relationships because they can't face the fact that their partner has fibromyalgia. They cannot cope with the stress, and face up to the fact that things will not be the same as they once were. It doesn't have to be that way.

Couples need to work on everything together, from health to finances; especially finances if one of you has to give up work.

Look at everything you can do together. It will not work if you both pull in different directions.

You loved your partner before fibromyalgia, so why not now? The person is still the same only with an illness. There is always help available to get things back on track.

It will not be easy and it will take time and a lot of effort. No one said living with fibromyalgia would be easy. You will need to look at life in a different light. You will see your partner struggle everyday with this illness. Listen to your partner about how they feel and learn all about the illness. You must take steps to work together, or it won't work at all.

Having fibromyalgia may drag you down to a state of despair. But you can have a normal healthy relationship that works for you, just by changing a few things. Open your mind to whatever comes up, and the challenges you may face together.

TAKE THE RIGHT

PLAN OF ACTION

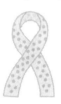

23

Getting The Most From Your Doctor

When I was first diagnosed with fibromyalgia, I was hoping that my doctor could fix me! I was broken and in bits with what was happening to me. I solely relied on my doctor to put things right. But this wasn't to be the case. I learnt I couldn't get the most from him! All I got was, 'I'm sorry. I cannot do anything for you. There is no cure for fibromyalgia. Take your medication. What do you want me to do?' This made me feel alone, utterly deflated, confused and I was left in tears after leaving the surgery.

One of the best things I did, was to find a doctor within the surgery who understood fibromyalgia. It is so easy for us to settle for the family doctor, but we all know that doctors vary from one to the other. We need one who understands the condition. Some doctors still have the notion that it is not real! In my opinion, a good doctor is one that has time for you, will listen to you, and will answer your question. He/she will explain why you need a new prescription and how the medication will help, and also suggest a new treatment for you. If your doctor isn't willing to answer all your questions, visit as many doctors in the surgery as you can. Do this until you find one that will help you?

As time went by, I wrote everything down. This covered everything from new symptoms, how I was feeling, and what part of my body was affected at that particular time. I handed the list to my doctor. I always practised what I wanted to say, but it never sounded right hence the list. I left the surgery no better than when I went in. We all know that each appointment is only 10 minutes. It is vital that you get as much as possible across. Remember, doctors are there to help you, to try to sort out any medical issues that you have. Believe it or not, doctors have a lot of help at their fingertips. Ask your doctor what treatments or courses are available in your area which may be beneficial to you. More to the point is what are you willing to try?

IT IS OK NOT TO BE OK,

AND TO ASK FOR HELP

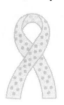

24

Never Stop Looking For Help

I was referred to many professionals and specialist doctors by my own doctor. Help is available. All you have to do is ask. Of course, this is my experience, not all doctors are the same. Some of you may have experienced what I have. But not all of you.

Quite often I hear people saying, 'But I don't have any support, not even my own family believes or supports me.' This is a real problem for some fibromyalgia sufferers.

From my experience, support is very much in demand. So many sufferers do not get the right support, and are, quite often left to deal with things on their own! It is sad to see a vast amount of people suffering with this condition without guidance and proper support. You CANNOT deal with fibromyalgia alone.

Just because your doctor is unable to do much for you, which is quite common, it's not the end! Never rely completely on just your doctor. There are other medical professionals who can help you. These are:

- Osteotherapists
- Occupational Therapists
- Physiotherapists
- Rheumatologists - doctors who deal with fibromyalgia
- Cognitive Behavioural Therapists
- Sleep Specialists
- Pain Therapists
- Mindfulness Therapy
- Neurologists
- Counsellors
- Alternative Health Practitioners: acupuncture, reiki etc.

All these professions have medical knowledge, some more than others, on how to help their fibromyalgia patients.

YOU CANNOT DEAL

WITH FIBROMYALGIA ALONE

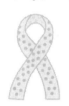

25

I`m In A Fibro Flare. What Helps Me?

When the symptoms of fibromyalgia begin to start acting up, it's often referred to as a fibro flare. This happens to sufferers on a regular basis.

What I have tried so far:

- Taking long hot baths in Epsom salts or Radox muscle soak crystals
- Rubbing in almond oil with marjoram, lavender and juniper oil on to the aching and painful joints. I also added drops of juniper, lavender and marjoram to bath water.
- Listening to music for distraction
- Taking stronger pain relief medication
- Using heat pads or hot water bottles on affected areas
- Relaxation techniques
- Diaphragm breathing exercises
- Improving sleep techniques
- Plenty of rest
- Learning from others

- Taking very slow walks down my street
- Taking up a new hobby for distraction
- Graded exercising
- Applying Tiger Balm on to affected areas
- Posture improvements
- Magnesium oil
- Aromatherapy
- Osteotherapists
- Physiotherapy
- Support groups

NOT EVERYTHING YOU MAY

COME ACROSS WILL HELP

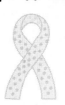

26

A New Hobby Helped

I had always had an interest in art, design and computer technology from an early age. I could never draw. I was useless at it, until that is, I began to understand computer graphics! One day, I downloaded a free trial of a computer drawing programme. I spent hours learning the package and it gave me something to focus on. When I felt tired, instead of taking an afternoon nap, I would get to grips with the software. Minutes became hours, and I didn't feel so tired anymore.

I heard that a friend of mine who used to do card making at home, was getting rid of some crafting materials. I asked her if I could have these materials and she said, 'Of course.' The next day she came around with four large boxes of crafting materials. I was astounded! She didn't want my money. I told her that once I got going I would make her a little something for her kindness and generosity.

Each day in between my goal setting routine, I started making cards. The aches and pains were still there, but because I was focused on something else, the symptoms didn't seem so bad. This was awesome! Every day I was designing and making cards. This really gave me a sense of achievement. I loved it! For once in a long time, I was beginning to feel happy. I started to buy more card making materials. I even started walking into town to my local craft shop. I struggled with the walking but I pushed through. When it got too much for me, my dad came and picked me up. Bless him! This was also getting me out of the house, which was good, because I was becoming a recluse. I made more of an effort than before. These crafting materials that I wanted gave me something to push for! As soon as I was in the house, I went into crafting mode. All sorts of ideas went through my mind.

I then thought, 'What about fibromyalgia awareness wallet cards?' I made these cards, handed them out to family and friends to explain the fibromyalgia syndrome. They went down very well, showing how this can affect each and every one of us.

I will NEVER stop my crafting or coming up with ideas to spread awareness of fibromyalgia. There is still not enough awareness, and everybody needs to know how fibromyalgia can destroy lives.

HAVING A HOBBY

REALLY HELPS

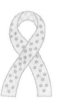

27

Symptom Diary

Halfway through my journey with fibro, I began to make a symptom diary.

I would write down what symptoms I was having, and what times of the day, how I was generally feeling, and what the weather was like - a cold or a hot day.

I did this with the food I was eating, just to see if food made a difference. This is a tricky one, as science hasn't yet proved to have any significance on how looking at your diet helps to improve fibromyalgia. But it was certainly worth noting.

Taking medication, could side-effects have an impact on how I felt and what symptoms I was experiencing?

I started writing every symptom that occurred over a period of 4 weeks:

Where was the pain located?

Arms	Legs	Shoulders
Ankles	Feet	Neck
Hips	Hands	Fingers
Jaw	Chest	Knees

How was I feeling? Were there any differences in my symptoms?

Stressed	Depressed	Anxious
Fatigued	Hot	Cold

What was the weather like on the day?

Hot	Cold

Including temperature and humidity

What was I eating and drinking?

Breakfast	Lunch
Dinner	Supper

What position was my body in?
Did my posture make any difference?

Sitting down	Lying down
Standing up	Kneeling down
Bending	

What was the severity of the pain?

- No pain
- Mild annoying pain
- Nagging uncomfortable pain
- Distressing miserable pain
- Intense dreadful pain
- Excruciating pain - worst possible

How often did the pain occur?
Did exercising contribute and bring on symptoms?

Pain	Fatigue	Breathlessness
Migraine	Dizziness	

Sleeping?

Was sleeping disturbed?
Did I sleep at all?
How many hours did I sleep?
Did my mattress, and how many pillows I had contribute?

Over the course of 4 weeks, I noticed a difference. Without writing it down, I wouldn't have taken any notice. I started to put things in motion from my symptom diary results. Over time I started to feel better. I identified my triggers, and how to manage them better. I would certainly recommend any fibromyalgia sufferer to do symptom diary. Identify your triggers and maybe you can try to change them - use the template above. There will be no two sufferers having the same results.

It's worth mentioning your symptom diary to your doctor. They may find alternative treatments that would benefit you. Having a symptom diary and showing it to my doctor paid off. I had another two diagnoses which contributed to my fibromyalgia symptoms. I wouldn't have known this without a symptom diary. As fibro covers an immense number of difficulties, you may find ways of coping better. Anything that helps is better than nothing.

A SYMPTOM DIARY:

IT MAKES SENSE

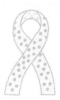

28

Learn To Say "NO"

Does this sound familiar! I was finding myself repeating so many apologies all the time. I felt guilty as I was the one everybody turned to if they needed help, or needed something done. I was always there to lend a hand when needed.

I now know that having and living with fibromyalgia limits you far beyond comprehension. We just cannot do what we used to. Do you find yourself constantly apologising ...

- I'm sorry, the kitchen looks like a bomb has hit it; I've not cleaned up.

- I'm sorry, I can't lend you money like I used to. I'm only on benefits.

- I'm sorry, I can't go out like I used to.

- I'm sorry, I can't be there for you if you need me.

- I'm sorry, I can't do these things like I used to.

- I'm sorry, I just can't do it ...

- I'm sorry ...

Why should we be apologising for having fibromyalgia. We never asked for it. We never wanted the limitations it brings.

I`M SORRY,

IT'S NOT MY FAULT

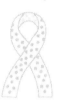

29

The Love Of My Family

My family understood and were behind me 100% as they had seen how this illness was affecting me on a daily basis; also physically, mentally and emotionally. All they could do was to try and understand what I was going through and be there for me in my hours of need.

My dad did all the running around: shopping, cooking, and cleaning. He did everything. He took me to the doctors and hospital when I needed to go. He took me to town and picked me up if I was in difficulty. Nothing was too much trouble. My mum always reassured me that I was going to be alright and allowed me to rest up. I could never have imagined that I would have to rely so much on my parents to take care of me at the age of 45. It's an awful feeling to have. It makes you feel like you're a burden, not just to your parents, but to your whole family and friends.

Mum and Dad took care of everything for me. I owe them so much. I love them both with all my heart.

IF OUR FAMILIES

DON'T UNDERSTAND,

THEN IT'S HARD FOR

ANYONE ELSE TO UNDERSTAND

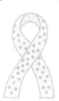

30

My Fifteen Minutes Of Fibromyalgia

1. The minute you're diagnosed, is the minute your whole life changes.

2. The minute you fall asleep, is the minute you're awake.

3. The minute you feel relaxed, is the minute you're tense.

4. The minute you feel warm, is the minute you sweat buckets.

5. The minute you move, is the minute you ache.

6. The minute you stand, is the minute you can't move.

7. The minute you feel OK, is the minute you could cry for no reason.

8. The minute you ache, is the minute you're in pain!

9. The minute you explain to friends, is the minute they disappear.

10. The minute you have to leave your job, is the minute the stress starts.

11. The minute you need help, is the minute where no one gives a damn.

12. The minute you take medication, is the minute the weight piles on.

13. The minute the pain starts, is the minute you feel you're in hell.

14. The minute you dream, is the minute the nightmares begin.

15. The minute we get the cure, is the minute we get our lives back!

THERE IS NEVER A MINUTE

WHERE FIBROMYALGIA

LEAVES YOU ALONE!

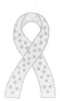

31

Myths & Misconceptions Of Fibromyalgia

Often I came across myths and misconceptions about how people see fibromyalgia. Below is just some of what I used to hear quite often. It's just so sad how people can judge one another without really having any idea of what fibromyalgia is and the impact it has on someone's health.

- You look fine, you must feel fine.
- If your pain were truly physically based, your mental state wouldn't affect your symptoms.
- If you are enjoying yourself, you must feel okay.
- Stress reduction techniques, such as meditation, are a cure for chronic pain.
- Depression results from a personality weakness or character flaw.
- And people who are depressed could snap out of it if they tried hard enough.
- Fibromyalgia isn't a real medical problem, "it's all in your head!"
- Change your diet; it will help you solve the pain.

- All you need is "rest" you will be okay tomorrow.
- If you can get dressed in a morning, you can go to work.
- Being home all day is a great lifestyle.
- You are just depressed.
- You just want to claim benefits and not go to work.
- Fibromyalgia doesn't exist, it's a made up illness.
- You need to get out of the house more.
- Your doctor has told you it's all in your head.
- Fibromyalgia is just a belief system.

Fibromyalgia is one of those conditions whereby, if you do not suffer from it, you will have no real comprehension about how it can be so debilitating.

WORDS CAN

HURT, TOO

32

Fibromyalgia Poems
by Shayne E Town

Pain, Pain, Pain

Fibromyalgia you're making it tough,
Please leave my life I've had enough!

For years you've made me sick and ill,
Suffering times with no magic pill.

The sun is shining the weather is sweet,
Time to crawl out of bed and on my feet.

The morning brings a sad day again,
Bringing more sickness and aching my brain.

Pain, Pain, Pain, oh, please no,
My little body is aching it's starting to show.

How can I take much more of this?
Please not to today and give me a miss.

As I sit writing this poem, the pain
And symptoms are starting I can feel them flowing.

Head is pounding beyond belief,
Why does it keep giving me so much grief?

What have I done to deserve this illness?
But each day I wake just brings more sickness.

As each day comes I will take it`s wrath,
Hoping I will get better and take a different path.

Where Do I Belong?

In my life you`re the one I thing I fear,
Living with pain, this you must hear.

Every day the pain will increase,
No life, No sleep, No peace.

I once had a life before fibromyalgia come along,
Now I shut my eyes, and think now where do I belong?

I wake up each day with things on my mind,
Only to struggle, this day will be another grind.

Now I hide, to where I think it`s safe,
Where no one knows about the pain that I have to face.

You look back on your life and think what I have done,
You`re losing yourself in who you`ve become.

It`s so sad that people often see you crying in pain,
Reaching out for help, but only to say you are lying again.

I don't worry too much, but a day will come,
When revenge will be given for the damage you`ve done.

I feel like the black skies of thunder,
Where is my life heading it makes me wonder.

What have I done to deserve this condition?
But one day it might just go into remission,
Where the pain won't strike,
So I can get on with my life.

33

My Ten Commandments

1. Thou shalt be of help to other sufferers.

2. Thou shalt find a hobby one is passionate about, and pursue it.

3. Thou shalt try and learn more about fibromyalgia.

4. Thou shalt assess thy diet, with added vitamins and minerals.

5. Thou shalt try at least 15 to 30 minutes daily exercise.

6. Thou shalt try and learn to say, 'No!'

7. Thou shalt not feel guilty in any way shape or form, for how fibromyalgia affects oneself.

8. Thou shalt make time for oneself.

9. Thou shalt be more considerate, gentle, loving and caring.

10. Thou shalt always try to be positive and hopeful for the future.

34
Stories From Fibromyalgia Sufferers

Housework

By Janet Ward

Housework is a word that covers a multitude of sins! We all hate doing it but feel good when it's been done. Everybody, man or woman, take pride in their homes, and rightly so. Nobody wants a dirty or messy home. A person with fibromyalgia feels the same.

Where shall I start? Cleaning can be really tiring—we all say that. People can say, 'But you've got a vacuum cleaner.' Maybe we have, but nobody sees us struggle. Using a light weight vacuum is just as heavy as a standard one if you have fibromyalgia.

Getting up can be a struggle to start with, then you look around and see that you need to do some cleaning. Out comes the Hoover, and then the fun starts. Plug in and off you go - hold on not so fast! A sufferer can't gallop through this like we used to. Yes we would like to, but we can't. Stop. Start. Stop. Start. If I had timed myself, you would be amazed cleaning an average sized room can take 20 minutes plus. This doesn't include polishing. This activity could take, again, up to 20 minutes. Why so long? I can hear people say. It hurts to stand up for too long. You get pelvic pain, and this is more common in women.

Washing up—this can be so tedious and tiring. Not everybody has a dish washer, and those that do, can have trouble loading. Bending to fill them cause's pain. If standing causes pain, get a stool and try that. This works to some extent, but you can't sit still (I know I can't) because you start aching, but you carry on regardless until you are finished. Then you sit down and recharge your batteries.

Let's go into bedroom next. Here the fun and games begin. Making your bed can cause pain. Straightening your sheet can cause pain because of your back. So what do you do? Sit on the bed and rumple the sheet so you have to pull that. Duvets, are, to coin a phrase, "a pain". Even the lightest tog can hurt to throw it on the bed. I have to pick mine up and pull it where I want it. Changing the bed becomes a massive feat. Gone are the days when you could put your duvet into a clean cover in minutes! These days it can take me up to 10 minutes.

Now to do the washing. Drag the wash basket from the bathroom to the kitchen. Once again, get a stool to sit on while you sort them out. Put the washing in the machine and select your temperature. I'm lucky, the temperatures I use most have been pre-programmed; all I have to is press buttons. However, some people suffer with turning knobs. Pegging the washing out is a No! No! I can't lift my arms high enough to peg them on the line or a rotary drier. I have to ask family members if they have time to help me. I have a tumble drier where the temperature that I use is left on, all I have to do is, again, touch buttons.

Ironing—this is done sat down. The ironing board set on its smallest height.

Recreation

By Janet Ward

Fibromyalgia sucks! How often have we either heard or said it. Fibromyalgia attacks our bodies. It wiggles its way inside you, and there it stays a life sentence! Let us sit down and transport ourselves back in time before this condition evaded our bodies.

I was the eldest of four children, but the only girl. I had to stick up for myself at an early age. We were lucky we lived close to a recreation ground (Goose Fair comes and sets up here) and would spend enjoyable afternoons there: having a rough and tumble, kick about with a football, playing on swings etc. on the park. We would also take ourselves to The Arboretum, look round, talk to the Parrot, have a picnic near the duck pond - these ducks were really well fed.

Time passed and I went to work. The company I worked for was great and I enjoyed the work. After time we held inter-departmental quizzes and spelling bees. It was all done in fun. I was working in the main sales department. We used to sit and talk at lunchtimes, and we talked about, and did get a netball team up. This was real fun and every Saturday we either trained or played a match. We had joined a league; it was competitive, but fun.

The years passed. I got married, still worked, but for a different company. We were members of the community centre. We held dances, games evenings and had a quiz team and travelled to different centres. This was all done for fun and a good time was had by all.

Time went by and unfortunately by husband died. I was left to bring up a small child on my own. My mum was in wheelchair and we would spend a lot of time with my mum. When we took her out, we either walked or caught a bus. I enjoyed the walking.

After a while, my best friend set me up on a blind date. Her friend had a brother and she set him up. It all went well and Alan travelled from Hull (where he came from) every weekend to be with me. After nearly a year, Alan moved in with me. The local pub we went to held quiz nights. These were great and we enjoyed them.

We both joined the local community centre, where I joined the darts team. We went all over Nottingham playing matches. This was really good fun, and at the end of season, we found out were top of the bottom league and we got a medal each.

Looking back I was really active. I was working and life was good.

All my recreation activities were group games. I know that I couldn't do any of them now that I have fibromyalgia. I am, however, walking small distances. I can't walk far because it hurts.

I know a lot of fellow fibromyalgia sufferers can't walk, but we can reflect and know what we did earlier has no impact with fibromyalgia. This condition leaves us bereft. Once it settles, it's here for good. All we can do is find some activity we can do, and show this illness we are fighting it.

Chronically Invisible

By Ella Cooper

I have always had problems with my joints and my back. My wrists and ankles were tender and weak, and I used to sprain them regularly. I went to physiotherapists, but I was just told, 'You probably are hyper mobile.' They told me this, without tests or assessments to prove this theory and rule out other conditions.

My knees used to swell regularly with no apparent reason. My back hurt if I did too much, such as lifting and cleaning. They used to hurt a lot more when I was cold. Doctors, physiotherapists and chiropractors put the pain down to my job. I am a Challenging Behaviour and Dementia Carer.

I paid £400.00 for chiropractor sessions and he was baffled as to why I wasn't improving. I didn't think the pain I felt in my wrists, ankles and back could be related.

I focussed on my back and went back to my GP. I was offered physiotherapy! They told me I should cut down my working hours as they couldn't find anything wrong. I had to take two weeks off work as the pain was getting unbearable. Once again I went back to my GP, I was told I was deficient in Vitamin D, and that's what was causing the pain. I took the tablets, but, no improvement.

I had to move in with my boyfriend. I'd found I was struggling to do everyday things. I struggled to put on my shoes, take a shower and even to sit up! When I moved, I also changed my doctor.

On my visit to see the new doctor, she looked through my notes, family history and tests. She's amazing, especially when she told me she knew what was wrong with me! This doctor didn't just assume I was too young to be suffering from anything serious.

I researched fibromyalgia, and it all made sense. My tiredness, which I hadn't really thought about, was because of fibromyalgia. I had thought my tiredness was all down to me, being unfit and a typical teenager sleeping all the time. I had also thought this tiredness was caused by being unable to sleep some nights because of the pain!

I have not had to change from full time work to go part time. I am still struggling, but, I have been told I'm fit for the job I'm doing ...

Connie's Constant Companion

By Connie Thompson

I was diagnosed with ME (Myalgic Encephalomyelitis) in 1991, after a string of different illnesses led to me being completely wiped off my feet. I became ill with pleurisy in April 1991, and just didn't get better. Then blood tests showed I had the Epstein Bar virus and the coxsackie virus.

I was laid up in bed, crawling on my hands and knees to go to the bathroom. I had no energy at all! Before this I was so active, always on the go, never stopping, even to draw breath. With three young children, there was so much to do and I couldn't do anything anymore.

At this time, we were living on the Isle of Lewis, and I was being sent away to hospital in Glasgow. I was having continuous tests and scans as I wasn't getting any better. My life, at this moment in time consisted of doctors, tests and medications, while my family could only sit and watch at the age of 28, me becoming like an old woman.

We moved to Edinburgh. My health wasn't good. I'd lost out on so much with my children because I couldn't do the things mums normally did with their children. This was all due to the chronic fatigue and pain all over my body. Sometimes I wished I could die as the pain was so bad. I had been diagnosed with osteoarthritis when I was 22. The pain I had then was totally different to the pain I was suffering now. I couldn't bear lights or sounds of any kind, as my head felt it would explode because of the pain. It couldn't have been easy living with me, because if they moved, I thought I was going to die, just because of the effect on my body.

My doctors referred me to a rheumatologist who told me I had fibromyalgia?! I had never heard of this, so he explained that the fatigue and pains were down to this illness. How I would never get better from this, but probably worse. I was to try and take each day at a time.

My whole world had come apart. I had, had plans to go back to college so I could retrain to have a career. I wanted some independence financially as well. All I could hear was I'd grow old and before my time! This was all down to having both ME and CFS. I am in constant pain 24/7, as if my body was on fire with the burning pain in my body. I have banged my head on the wall, just to see if the pressure of these constant headaches, would stop. Pressure behind my left eye was so severe, it felt like my eye might pop and stop the pain, but it doesn't.

The feeling of being freezing cold constantly, having the heating on full blast and everyone around me is stripping off, because the house was too hot for them. Chronic insomnia dominates my life, as I can't sleep. The slightest noise has me jumping out of my skin. I have a fan on every time I go to bed, so the white noise drowns out any other noise. Blackout blinds on the bedroom window wherever I go. I can't bear light of any kind because of the pain I feel from these lights.

This illness has ruined my life in so many ways. It's robbed me of my self-esteem, confidence, ability and me being me. I can't do things that my family and friends want me to do. This illness is invisible and they can't see "my constant companion", and they don't fully understand how I feel.

In the past two and a half years, I've had two major breakdowns because of the way this illness makes me feel. I feel useless, worthless, a waste of time and resources.

It breaks my heart to hear my now grown up children say, 'We can only remember you mum, as not being well and not doing things with us because of this.' I have tried to remind them of all I used to do with them.

I feel quite robbed by this illness, as it has taken so much away from me in every aspect of my life.

Fibromyalgia Warrior

By Jules Allen

When asked to talk about my battle with fibromyalgia, I am perturbed at where to start. It seems to have been a part of my life forever.

I was always more tired than my friends, even at school. I always put this down to not being athletic or the sporty type. As I reached my 20's this started to be an issue. I seemed to be in pain for no apparent reason at all. I wasn't just tired, but exhausted!

I was a mum to three before I was 30. Each time I went to the doctors I was told, "that's just the way it is!" or, "get some more sleep!" The worst of it was being told it was in my head! I started to believe them, I mean, these are doctors, right? You trust them, and they will always tell you the truth.

I tried pick me up tonics, vitamins and herbal remedies, but nothing helped. I would go back go back to the doctors from time to time, in the hope that the bloods would show something was; but they didn't. I just pumped more pain killers into my body and got on with it.

Let me fast forward to 2007. I am now 37 and have moved from my home town of Birmingham to Hampshire. I went to see my new GP for an examination and to go over my medical history. This day changed my life in many ways. We did the usual, chatted about the births of my children, my family history, blah, blah, blah. Then I mentioned this severe pain I was in and how my husband helped me to get out of bed on a daily basis. My GP looked at her screen. There was a deadly silence, and then the printer powered up. She handed me some papers with the heading "fibromyalgia".

After a brief chat, she told me to go away, read the information, and come back tomorrow. In a slight daze. I left the surgery and went home. Reading through this information was like reading my life story. All of this made sense to me. Going back the next day, I felt almost lighter; it wasn't in my head; I wasn't making it up. It was real and the relief was immense.

Don't get me wrong, it hasn't been plain sailing. I have seen doctors who don't believe this condition exists. They have told me I'm like this because I'm overweight. My GP has stood by me every step of the way. I know how very lucky I am to have such a supportive and helpful Health Care Practitioner. I can go to my GP with some research I have done, and, if it is safe to do so, she'll let my try pretty much everything.

When it all sank in, I was almost bitter that I, finally, had an answer. It was still something some people still believed it was in the patient's head. Why should I have to convince people I have an illness?

I will break it down to the parts that had I feel fibromyalgia has had the biggest impact on my life:

Family:

My family have been amazing—my kids know if I am in flare-up, and do all they can go help me. My husband struggles seeing me in pain, but he knows what I need, and how to deal with me. I feel guilty when I have to miss things: football matches, golf tournaments or a class assembly. These are the times it breaks my heart and I feel sorry for myself.

Friends:

Well this is a tricky one, because when you have fibromyalgia you do have to cancel plans, and that is hard for some people to understand. They assume you will let them down and even fall out when you can't make a birthday night out. I had to learn the hard way—'those who mind don't matter, and those who do matter don't mind!'

Work:

I had to give up my cleaning business which I had built up from scratch. It was all mine and I was devastated to give it all up. Physically I couldn't do this anymore. After attending an assessment with the DWP I was deemed unfit for work completely, and was put into the ESA support group.

I don't go down that easy, so off I went to see my trusty GP and said, "Right what can we do?" We tried all sorts of medication and finally found a combination that works for me; nine years since I was first diagnosed.

As well as fibromyalgia, I also suffer with IBS, general anxiety, panic attacks, adenomyosis and rheumatoid arthritis in my knees. It's a challenge most days, but I will say now, I'm not a victim—I am a warrior of fibromyalgia. You can exercise as it can have a positive effect, if you build up gently. It doesn't have to stop you doing anything you set your mind on.

I love nothing more than proving medical science wrong. Keeping up to date with research out there, finding people who suffer as well.

I have good days and bad days, but, I am eating well, walking when I can and taking my medication to at least allow me to enjoy my family and friends. A bad day is just that—a bad day, not a bad life.

How My Life Changed

By Tracey Crookes

Seven years ago I was planning my wedding. I decided to join a gym and buy a Wii Fit as well. All young girls want to look good on their special day.

I started to get pains in my hips. Rather than go to the doctors I tried over the counter creams and pain relief. This didn't seem to help so I made an appointment with my GP. He sent me for X-Rays and was so sure they would come back normal. I got my results and was told "wear and tear", nothing can be done only pain killers and creams.

I carried on working my three jobs as well as caring for my partner (now my husband). Things weren't getting any better, so I went back to the doctors. This time I was given more cream. He told me to keep a diary, because I was getting pain in other parts of my body; and see him in two weeks. I made an appointment but my doctor was on leave, so I saw a locum. By this time, I was struggling to walk. I explained what was wrong and showed her by diary. Well, she said she knew what was wrong with me. I was told I had something called fibromyalgia, but she wanted it confirmed. This doctor referred be to see a rheumatologist, and it was a long time waiting for an appointment.

When I went to see the rheumatologist, I told her what was going on. She ran some blood tests and examined me. When I went back for the results she confirmed fibromyalgia and ME. I never thought that fibromyalgia would change my life, but it has. I used to see friends and go out. If I go out now it's to the hospital and doctor appointments.

I am in pain, and tired all the time. I have illnesses caused by fibromyalgia; and can't have the life I had before and it leaves me isolated. Friends have been lost because they don't understand. My independence has gone because I can't do things all in one go like the housework, so I either have help or do things over a few days. I get frustrated because once I could clean the house all in one go and not be in pain. Now, any kind of cleaning or cooking causes pain because I can't stand for long periods. I never thought that at 30 years old, my life would change so much.

13 Stone Lighter, But Crippled By The Tin Man

By Robert Fraser

I'm 45 this year and have had fibromyalgia for ten years now. Two possible causes of my fibromyalgia are - the weight loss surgery in 2005, and the infection that nearly killed me in hospital! And a few months after the Hep B injections whilst working for a sanitation company.

Then, one Boxing Day, I became the Tin Man. I seized up solid and was bedridden for six weeks. After home visits from my GP, and an ambulance to take me to hospital, I received a massive dose of liquid steroid. This got me mobile again, but only to a fraction of my normal self. I literally went from being an EX 28 stone bloater to a 15 stone pain ravaged cripple and have been ever since.

What followed was a diagnosis for acute seronegative arthritis and now, fibromyalgia: both life changing and painful debilitating conditions. I applied for DLA and was awarded it after a GP who worked for ATOS, said he knew I was genuine after 30 seconds.

Life is intolerable now! I get frequent flare-ups, constant pain, and the medication is pathetically useless. The welfare system that is causing great personal anguish to me and many more sufferers.

I have just managed to keep working 30 hours a week, but at what cost to me, both physically and emotionally.

Two more points: a state sanctioned campaign, run by private companies who want to rob me of my lifetime DLA award. This has caused me frequent stress which aggravates all my conditions by making me apply for PIP. And the only medication that really helps is not legal in the UK. We (UK), are only just starting to wake up and debate the legislation of medical use cannabis. The UK now, as usual, lags behind twenty US states and at least twenty countries: Canada, Portugal, Holland, Spain, Denmark, Uruguay, Mexico, to name a few.

Change Of Life

By Linda Morris Ellard

My name is Linda Morris Ellard. My maiden name was Codona, and my Dad was related to the Fair Folk. Some of his ancestors belonged to the Circus.

I had a happy childhood, and as the eldest of three children, I was very active and good at sports and art. I left school at fifteen and throughout my adult life enjoyed a very active and successful career. I was a nurse, and a support learning assistant right up to the age of 60. I have never been unemployed.

As a member of several running groups, my husband and I ran three times a week. Life for us was full and exciting. I felt confident and enjoyed lots of hobbies. I studied for the ministry and also worked for the church for fourteen years. This was as well as a full time job in two special needs schools. During this time in the schools, I was found to be very flexible and enjoyed great success working with specialist teachers. The art room was my specialism for five years, and the swimming pool was my base for two years. I also specialized in the domestic science classes for two years. As you can see, I was flexible enough to work anywhere in the schools.

When I reached the age of 58, I started to experience health issues that seemed to defy any normal explanation. I had flu like symptoms, but they lasted too long and normal treatments made no change to how exhausted and sore I felt. Although it felt like flu, I had no high temperature, and I honestly thought I was malingering.

No matter what I did, and as a nurse I knew what to do. This constant exhaustion and physical pain that was widespread, and stopped me sleeping at night just got worse. I was signed off work for more than six months; and I was becoming paranoid. The GP was treating me for SAD (seasonal affective disorder), so I took the tablets and hoped for the best.

Eventually, I found working with the children painful. I couldn't run after them like I could before. It seemed I had ulcer symptoms, and IBS, not to mention severe migraine headaches which lasted three days. These could be triggered by movement of the car, and light flickering of buildings.

I was also apologizing, feeling as if someone had pulled the plug on me. My energy levels dropped considerably. I felt changed, no longer me, but I kept trying to reach my goals.

Towards the end of 2010, I was referred to a rheumatologist who diagnosed me with fibromyalgia. I had never heard of this before. My sister, from America, sent me all the books she could on this condition. Then I was referred to a pain clinic, which helped me at the time. The biggest mistake was the medication which was specific, but, this condition seemed to affect every part of my body. If sleepless was the main problem, medication might need to be increased.

The pain was widespread and physio wasn't really helpful; I wanted the old me back. Fibromyalgia has now changed me completely. It's like a death sentence—the old you is gone. You can no longer do the things you took for granted.

So, because of fibromyalgia, I retired when I was 60, and started learning to live with the new person I had become. I had to pace myself, find different work; voluntary that I could do that would allow for flare ups, and I had to find a self-help group that would make me feel valued and positive about things I could do. I saw myself as a work in progress - not a failure! Fibro Flare Magazine and Fibro Flare Sufferers of the UK have been a life line to me and given me back my sanity.

Between 2013 and 2014, I tried Mickle Therapy, which was an eye opener for me. It isn't a cure, but it helped me change my perspective, organise my life better, and challenge those who were negative influences in my life, and helped me to be the real me.

Like the Fibro butterfly, in a lovely shade of purple, I was changed! Not the menopause, but after a little pause, I accepted I had changed. I was still a work in progress, I didn't have to say goodbye to the old me. I am still here, somewhere.

Life After Work

By Beth Urmston

I am now 58 and first had symptoms of fibromyalgia at the age of 7. However these were flares, and for the most part I contrived to live a normal life.

I worked for thirty-five years but, due to the fibromyalgia being constant from 2007; I was forced to give up work in 2009.

This was totally devastating for me. The previous eighteen months had been extremely stressful, in part due to the fact I did not have a diagnosis. The manager did not believe I needed any adjustments as it was all in my mind!

For three years, I lived in a bubble of existence, until one of my carers suggested I try Facebook. I came across a fibromyalgia group and discovered that fibromyalgia wasn't just something that happened to me, or even a few people. Research showed there are millions of people also diagnosed with fibromyalgia.

It was then I had the idea to produce a magazine. The first issue went out in May 2014 and two years on, it is stronger than ever. All the work is done by volunteers - all fibromyalgia patients. This has given purpose to my life, the magazine and raising awareness.

Helping to support those who need it, and the discovery that children as young as three are suffering with fibromyalgia symptoms, motivates me to do whatever I can to give them all a better future: one where more people will be aware of the incapacitating, disabling affect this chronic condition has on lives, not only those with fibromyalgia, but families and close friends.

Fibromyalgia And Me

By Ian Hydon

I have officially had fibromyalgia for five years now, plus other chronic conditions as well. My beloved Mum, who was my rock and my world passed away in 2011. This happened a couple of weeks before I was diagnosed with fibromyalgia.

It took many years of going back and forth to the doctors and other specialists, before a rheumatologist eventually diagnosed fibromyalgia.

2011 and most of 2012 were awful for me! This was mainly because of my mum passing and me having fibromyalgia and severe osteoporosis diagnosed.

Then in June 2012, I was dealt another blow. The company where I'd given ten years of loyal service, announced the team was going to be disbanded—the work was going out of the country. We were given six weeks' notice. What made this worse was, that after thirteen months or so of not being able to work because of my mum, and the pain of the fibromyalgia, I was really ready to go back to work.

Whilst the nation celebrated the London 2012 Olympics, I was contemplating how on earth, with the pain of fibromyalgia and my exhaustion as well, how would I get another job? We are now at Easter 2016, and I am still wondering.

However, my fibromyalgia experience has made me even more empathic than I was before. I have been doing a whole series of voluntary work in the local community and also online.

The community work includes helping to support the elderly and the lonely. I know what that's like—being alone with chronic health conditions; every minute of every day.

I am also very active online, particularly with a number of fibromyalgia, CFS (Chronic Fatigue Syndrome) support groups. One Facebook fibromyalgia group is called 'Fibromites with Hope'. I took this group over as owner, moderator and prime admin on Christmas Day 2013. We had 590 members. As I write this at Easter 2016, we are now just short of 3000 members! A fivefold increase.

I love helping others who, like me are living with chronic pain and the tiredness of fibromyalgia. I have also been researching information for people, and am there to support them and be supported in return.

If you have been diagnosed with fibromyalgia, or any chronic pain condition and would like to join, you are most welcome.

I aim to spread awareness to the disbelieving world of what fibromyalgia is like. One day you may be able to do a lot; other days you are so tired and in great pain.

Some doctors still disbelieve us, and some think we are imagining things. Fibromyalgia has been recognized since the 1970's by the World Health Organisation as being a chronic condition.

I do try to get out every day, at least to go for a walk. I love nature. I am most relaxed the countryside. My fibromyalgia often dictates how much energy I have each day.

Well, this is my story. I hope it helps others - because you are not alone in living with fibromyalgia. There are lots of other people out there, something like 1 in 50 of the UK have it. Unfortunately it is for life.

My Fibromyalgia

By Cheryl Gomery

I'm going to tell you a secret - I'm fake! I'm 39 and try to be upbeat, positive and happy, but I can't. I live with my partner and daughter. In truth they are my carers, even though I try to be independent. I was never going to take fibromyalgia lightly, for various reasons.

I am an insulin dependent diabetic, have chronic pain syndrome, fibromyalgia. Chronic fatigue, depression, anxiety and acrophobia. They have also said lupus, but this hasn't been confirmed. Most days I'm confined to my bedroom, it's like prison! I think I have been in full flare since 2014.

All of my problems started when I was in a car accident in December, 2013. I experienced swollen joints, muscle spasms and extreme neck pain. X-Rays showed a break in my neck. They weren't sure about this; it could have been earlier. My GP is really supportive, but only works part-time.

I saw the rheumatologist—who was submissive and rude, and

told me to lose weight and all my problems would go. I lost some weight and guess what? Yes, the pain was still there and with a vengeance!

I was still positive to the outside world, wasn't leaving the house much, and still spent most of my time in the bedroom. Although I was hiding away, I was still posting positive posts on Facebook. My family really believed what I posted.

I was having a horrible time at work. I had a boss who didn't like me. My stress levels were really high. Some of my family had health problems. When depression set in, I was signed off work. I had meetings with the crisis team, but that didn't help—more tablets.

My dad passed away in 2014, and I fell out with some family members, and this still hasn't healed fully. It had a massive impact on my health. I tried different pain killers. I'm on quite strong oxycodone and a morphine patch. My skin was itching - this is called allodynia, a side effect of opiate pain killers.

My family questioned whether I really was ill as I kept posting positively on Facebook. I was only letting those close to me know just how vulnerable I was. I tried to explain but, some people only believe what they want to.

Over time, different anti-depressants were tried. I had bad reactions to some of these, so I went back on Prozac. I'm still taking a multitude of medication. I hate it all, but you just have to keep on taking them.

Fibromyalgia gives different guises, no two people are the same. I now get TMJD (temporal mandibular jaw disorder) through grinding my teeth. Many GPs dismiss this saying you're too young, just add this to your list of ailments.

I had to give up work because I couldn't do it properly. My doctor signed me off as unfit for work. I returned after a year off. I was expected to know all the changes despite not being there.

In 2015, I was so stressed out about leaving the house, feeling like I did. I kept falling asleep at my desk and slept lots. So I decide to cut my losses and give up work on amicable terms.

I got terrible headaches, treated as a sinus problem. However, it was another sign of fibromyalgia. I am not making tears so I use saline drops now. I've always had problems swallowing and digesting food. I have IBS and colitis. I don't eat much, but I'm still overweight.

I did a pain relief course. Some things helped, some didn't. I stayed in touch with some people on the course and they helped me put things into perspective. Looking at Facebook groups, you realise you aren't alone; other people suffer as well. Thinking about the past and present caused a catastrophic mental health issue. The mental health team gave me advice.

In 2015, I spent the latter end inside the house, unable to go out.

I can't go up and down stairs easily and have trouble getting in the shower and bathing myself. I had acupuncture and this had good and bad effects. I still post happy thoughts on Facebook.

I exercise most days, when I can cope with it. Fibromyalgia has lost the old me and many aspects of my life. It has changed the way I see the world, and realise other people are the same as me. I'm frustrated and feel I am not living, but existing. I feel like a burden. I've been diagnosed with having bulimic tendencies and life is a constant battle.

Guess what? I will go on Facebook in an effort to gain some sort of normality. I'm not sure I miss the old me; I think she carried on regardless, and did as she was told. That isn't me, and if I want to post things on Facebook on a day that I feel crap and tell everyone, then I will.

My Fight Against Fibromyalgia

Esther Whitwam

I miss my life before fibromyalgia. I was a bubbly, happy outgoing teenager. Since I was 15 I was training to be a fire fighter, going in once a week for training. I didn't know anything was going to change, and I wouldn't have a normal life. Then at the age of 16, I started having knee problems. The doctor said I had no cartilage and I was on crutches for six weeks.

At the age of 19, I was out with my boyfriend, and suddenly I lost complete feeling in my leg. We went to A&E. I had an X-ray, CT scan and a MRI and other tests. They couldn't find anything wrong, but then they did a nerve test and, at the age of 19 I was diagnosed with fibromyalgia.

How would you describe the pain and symptoms faced regularly? The pain is awful. Waking up is agony—sore and weak muscles. One day tolerable, one day excruciating. My symptoms are:

- Fatigue
- Extreme back ache, sometimes it feels like its locking

- Tingling in legs, hands feet
- Shaky
- Stomach pains
- Mood swings
- Depression
- Sleepless nights
- Restless leg syndrome, frequent muscle pain and spasms
- Confusion or Fibro Fog
- Sensitivity to pain
- Chest pain.

My life has changed dramatically since my diagnosis. I can't go out with my friends. I'm in a wheelchair and my husband has to come along! A simple five minute walk is agony. Everyday I'm stuck in the same four walls—it's really hard, because you want to go out but you can't.

I'm quite lucky really; all my friends understand what I'm going through. They help my husband with chores, wheelchair pushing and keeping me upbeat.

Fibromyalgia can affect relations and relationships. After my diagnosis I gave my boyfriend the chance of walking away, and I wouldn't judge him. Instead, he asked me to marry him, and said he'd always be here for me, no matter what! At this point I knew everything would be ok. We've had our ups and downs, when I thought I was just a burden. He does so much for me that I question if I am holding him back. In fact, I know he wants me, to help me, otherwise he would have walked when he had the choice.

We are trying for a baby; we both want children. This isn't easy for us as there's been so much planning. It could cause me more pain and I may have to come off my medications.

Life Before Fibromyalgia

By Chelle Priestley

OK - so my life before fibromyalgia? I had become less active due to having Meniere's disease, but still managed to be fairly active. Slowly but surely, everything started to be a struggle. My left knee started hurting first. I went on a diet, but this didn't help. When I started having pains in my fingers and hands I went to my doctor who, after examining me, said it was probably fibromyalgia.

I lost my grandad who was my absolute hero. The stress sent me into depression and anxiety—so more medication. I was constantly tired, and I don't mean from too many late nights. This tiredness was nothing like I'd felt before. I started going to bed when I wasn't working, when I was, fibro fog made my job very difficult. The pains made it difficult moving around the school, and I was signed off. After eighteen months I lost my job. So I now found myself dealing with a new illness, no job and not being as active as I was.

Constant exhaustion made me feel a crap mother, sister and friend. Fibromyalgia stole the really active and happy go lucky person I once was. This has left me an overweight, miserable recluse. I spend so much time at the doctors I ought to have my own chair. Each day is dictated by my medications, my diary, and my appointments as I never know how I'm going to feel. So I don't make plans.

Both my doctor and rheumatologist think that if I lost weight, I would be cured! There isn't a diet out there that I haven't tried. All that happens is I keep gaining weight, which makes me more depressed.

I can't open bottles and jars, and struggle to write as my fingers lock up. Sleep is something I crave and I'm not sure I will ever get it.

I just pray that either a cure is found, or I don't get any worse. My normal life has gone, but I still grieve it.

Fibromyalgia And Me

By Pam Wooller

I first started with fibromyalgia in my mid 30's. I had a lot of back pain, and aching legs. This, I put down to an accident at work. I started physiotherapy and specialist groups but they didn't help.

Luckily my children were growing up, so didn't need as much "Mum, can you do?" and things were less physical. I did however, move to an office job. Thankfully they were understanding and provided me with a decent chair for support. As time went on I learnt to accept the pain, but then, the tiredness and forgetfulness began; and the aching was getting increasingly more frequent.

My mum kept saying I had fibromyalgia like her! Hey—I wasn't having any of it. I mean, she's older and this was her illness. I didn't know what was happening to her, and by the time I did, it was too late. I went to my GP who did blood tests and the diagnosis was hypothyroidism. I had just turned 40 and my doctor started me on thyroxine and had to have yearly blood tests.

It continued like this until five years ago. I lost my mum and they suspected her illness was genetic. My symptoms were worsening. I put this down to stress.

I went to my GP and was sent for a test, and yes, unfortunately, I have the same condition— haemochromatosis. There is no medication for this. 500ml of your blood is taken and thrown away: until you are at a set level. For a normal person this would be anaemia. I decided to mention these symptoms, as they cross over a lot with fibromyalgia; a lot of people can be misdiagnosed.

It's now June 2013, the pain was absolutely unbearable. My breaking point was I couldn't pick my eight week old baby up! I literally couldn't bear moving my fingers. I felt like I was on fire— but a cold fire.

Back to my GP who suggested fibromyalgia. Reluctantly I agreed to the tender point test. I remember that day so well, one of the points hurt that much I yelped, jumped and laughed. It was ridiculous it hurt that much! I was told I scored 14 out of 19. She put me on Co-Codamol and low dose amitriptyline; nothing stronger as I had my daughter to care for.

I went back to work in April 2014. The pain was there nearly every day. My chair was broken and the desk low. I simply couldn't think because of fibromyalgia. I had to go on sick leave and the doctor changed my medication and referred me to a rheumatologist. I saw him in November. He asked questions, examined me, and took bloods. I was then told I had widespread osteoarthritis and fibromyalgia, and to keep active or I'd end up in a wheelchair. He was so dismissive, offered no support, just that my GP would get a letter.

However, as I was still off work, Occupational Health were now involved (I worked for the NHS). The consultant was nice and suggested hydrotherapy, a change in medication and office equipment that was more suitable. My medication was changed. Gabapentin made me feel worse. I felt dizzy and washed out and gained weight. Hydrotherapy would leave me wiped out and bed ridden. My little girl needed me.

Work was no better: no equipment. So Occupational Therapy suggested my medication be changed and they would write my manager to chase the equipment I needed. Honestly, work went from bad to worse, and I handed my notice in after various meetings and being demoted.

Before I got worse with this, I was at the gym three times a week. My husband and I rode bikes and loved dancing. I really loved decorating, but going up ladders is now a no-no. I've lost friends through cancelling dates at the last minute. I constantly feel like I had a session at the gym. I can't sleep properly as bright lights wake me up. I have to plan really carefully if Mia, my daughter, has an activity to go to. It's not her fault I have this condition. I've explained to friends and family how I feel and have to cancel dates. I've now learnt to dance in my wheelchair.

This illness has isolated me, took my self-esteem, made me feel embarrassed because people can't see what's wrong, and gives depression and a whole lot of anger to be contained. I feel guilty about my mum and the only support is from other people who also have it.

I am grateful for the online support group, which the author of this runs. It's the only place where I can vent, support and be supported.

Living In Hell With Fibromyalgia

By Donna Turner

On the 13th December 2015, I was diagnosed with fibromyalgia. It has made my life and health a living hell. I have not been able to keep up the pace I was used to before fibromyalgia.

The one thing about fibromyalgia support groups I am in, is getting to know people who have this condition, and making so many new friends, sharing thoughts and crossing information.

Since having fibromyalgia, I have noticed that all but a few of my friends have disappeared from my life because of it. They do not understand the condition. They have no idea how I suffer day in and day out. This doesn't bother me because, the one true, loving, caring and understanding person who I have had the pleasure of talking to is the author of this book. He completely understands me because he has been, the one true friend I can turn to and trust. He's always around to provide support and advice when I need it.

The feeling of having support, and knowing you can turn to

somebody for support is amazing. I know I'm not alone in my battle with this chronic condition which only sufferers seem to understand.

It Hurts, Like Living In Hell

By Andrea Raso

I was diagnosed in 2009 and I was taking care of my mum, who was going through cancer treatments. I started to feel ill: pain, horrible fatigue and weakness. I kept this to myself and waited till her treatments were almost over. It got so bad I thought I had MS.

When I was diagnosed my life instantly changed overnight. I couldn't do the things I did before fibromyalgia. I was only 41 and instantly became 81. Everything changed!

My sleeping became affected, where I wasn't sleeping for weeks on end.

My fibromyalgia has progressed over the years and has, basically ruined my life. I don't feel "normal" anymore. Arguments with my fiancée became regular because fibromyalgia stopped me doing things and going places. I have missed so many important events and memories.

I've become a shell of the person I once was - I have lost friends. They do not understand how fibromyalgia devastates me on a regular basis. The ones who have stuck around have distanced themselves.

I now live in constant fear that I will end up totally alone and in a wheelchair. I have never been one to take medications or over the counter drugs for fibromyalgia symptoms or the pain; due to sensitivities to medication, so I suffer more!

The bottom line is. I feel like a waste. I have a degree in Social Work, but feel I can't use my skills anymore. Fibromyalgia has taken everything from me!

The author of this book has been brilliant to me. Always there for a chat day or night. He's been the only one who has stood by me in difficult times and has helped pull me through when days seemed too much for me. This man has literally saved my life more than once. He is my angel and saving grace. I could never repay him for all he has done for me. This has all made our bond stronger; we have an extremely close friendship.

I consider him one of my best friends. I love him and ... thank you!

35

What Does The Future Hold?

Don't ever think that because we don't hear of new drugs or treatments we will be left to suffer alone. It couldn't be further from the truth. The future is bright for fibromyalgia sufferers.

Living with the pain and symptoms of this condition is very frustrating, but will be significantly changing in the future. Medical research has proven that fibromyalgia is not all in your head, but is, in fact a serious condition to live with. A prodigious amount of clinical trials have led to a greater recognition of fibromyalgia by doctors and the general public.

The future holds a lot of hope as scientists are looking at new treatments, not just for the pain we experience, but also new therapy for the symptoms we are experiencing. Research is also focusing on genetic studies. A part of the brain called the insular, or insular cortex and insular lobe may be involved in the pathophysiology of fibromyalgia.

Research studies are also underway looking at new ways to

provide new drugs without the major side effects. Scientists have yet to prove the exact cause of fibromyalgia. However, new brain imaging studies have found abnormalities in patients with fibromyalgia. They are looking at ways in which the brain responds to pain caused by this condition is proving critical for future studies.

Fibromyalgia Patient Education Programmes are underway and available worldwide. More studies are also being funded. There is still a long way to go.

In respect to all research there is still HOPE every day, certainly the future looks bright in treating fibromyalgia.

THE PAIN WE SUFFER IS REAL,

AND SO IS HOPE

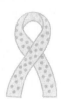

36

Conclusion

Don't ever be misled by others who say "they have the cure", or claim, "to have been cured". A cure does NOT exist, and if that's the case they never had fibromyalgia in the first place.

I'm always trying to find new ways of dealing with and fighting fibromyalgia. We cannot allow this condition to take over our lives.

Fibromyalgia has certainly taught me how to become more compassionate, and show empathy towards others. As a sufferer I know exactly what you are feeling, and going through daily. I have learnt how to challenge myself.

I want to raise more awareness of this condition. Fibromyalgia will destroy your life if you let it. Challenging yourself will enable you to make improvements to your life.

I hope that by reading my book, and what fibromyalgia has put me through, you will have a better understanding of this illness.

You will see what can be achieved with a little effort, and what changes you can make to improve your life.

You do not have to suffer in silence. Remember you are not alone in the battle with fibromyalgia. Be strong and stay strong.

All the best to you and your future.

S E Town

37

Fibromyalgia Notebook

Steps Forward

Remember: Taking little steps forward may help you achieve your aims and goals in the future.

- Try and think of three realistic goals that you would consider achieving
- Pick one of these that you need to focus on
- Think about what you might need, or change in order to achieve this:

1 _____

2 _____

3 _____

_____

_____

_____

_____

_____

What benefits are you noticing from exercising?

- A little improvement
- No improvement
- Makes me feel worse

_____

_____

_____

_____

What techniques are you already using?

- Exercise
- Complementary therapies
- Pacing
- Relaxation with or without music

_____

_____

_____

_____

_____

How often are you exercising?

_____

_____

_____

_____

Are there any other treatments you would like to try?

_____
_____
_____
_____
_____
_____
_____

What are your main triggers?

_____
_____
_____
_____
_____
_____

Any changes in diet?

_____
_____
_____
_____
_____
_____

What have you changed for the positive?

_____

_____

_____

_____

_____

_____

_____

What do you want to change?

_____

_____

_____

_____

_____

_____

_____

_____

What's working for you?

_____

_____

_____

_____

_____

REMEMBER THE

SYMPTOM DIARY: CHAPTER 27

38

Useful Addresses (UK)

Fightback4Justice
Michelle Cardno
Suite 21/22 Ela Mill
Cork Street
Bury
BL9 7DU
Manchester
Tell: 0161 672 7444 (General Enquiries/Advice)
Tell: 0161 667 5258 (Advocacy Help (Form Filling and Booking
for Form Filling)
Website: www.fightback4justice.co.uk

Fibromyalgia Action UK
Studio 3007, Mile End Mill
12 Seedhill Road
Paisley PA1 1JS
Tell: 0844 887 2444 (general)
Tell: 0844 826 9022 (Fax)
Website: www.fmauk.org

Fibroduck Foundation
Unit 191 Blackpool Selfstore,
Tellcom Business Centre,
20 Clifton Road, Blackpool
FY4 4QA
www.fibroduckfoundation.com
Email: fibroduckfoundation@gmail.com
Tel: 07739 644164

IBS Network
Unit 1.12, SOAR Works
14 Knutton Road
Sheffield S5 9NU
TEL: 0114 272 3253
Website: www.theibsnetwork.org

Employment and Support Allowance (ESA)
Tel: 0800 055 6688
Textphone: 0800 023 4888
Welsh language telephone: 0800 012 1888
Monday to Friday, 8am to 6pm
Website: www.gov.uk/employment-support-allowance/how-to-claim

DWP - Personal Independence Payment claims (PIP)
Telephone: 0800 917 2222
Textphone: 0800 917 7777
Monday to Friday, 8am to 6pm
Website: www.gov.uk/pip/how-to-claim

Bladder and Bowel Foundation
SATRA Innovation Park
Rockingham Road
Kettering
Northants NN16 9JH
Tel: 01536 533 255 (General enquires)
Tel: 0845 345 0165 (helpline)
Website: www.bladderandbowelfoundation.org

Citizens Advice
This advice applies to England
Contact Consumer line if you're in Northern Ireland.
Call the helpline Citizens Advice consumer helpline:
03454 04 05 06
Textphone: 18001 03454 04 05 06
Monday to Friday, 9am to 5pm
To contact a Welsh-speaking adviser: 03454 04 05 05
Textphone to contact a Welsh-speaking adviser:
18001 03454 04 05 05
Website: www.citizensadvice.org.uk

39

Social Media Support Groups

Fibromyalgia UK Awareness Fighters
Shayne Elliott Town
https://www.facebook.com/groups/Fibromyalgiaukawareness

Fibromyalgia Family – You`re Not Alone
Julie Bexley & Theresa Miller
https://www.facebook.com/groups/1645989475667771

Fibromites with Hope
Ian Hydon
https://www.facebook.com/groups/277430278984970

Fibroflare magazine
Beth Urmston
https://www.facebook.com/groups/Fibroflare
http://pubhtml5.com/bookcase/kgem

Fibromyalgia Support Group U.K (PHOENIX)
Robert Fraser
https://www.facebook.com/groups/Phoenixfibro

Tameside Fibro & CFS/ME – Private
Yvonne Buckingham
https://www.facebook.com/groups/179007298904884/

UK Fibromyalgia and Chronic Fatigue Syndrome
Janine Truslove
https://www.facebook.com/groups/988833847808842

Fibromyalgia Nite Owls
Marian Boyd
https://www.facebook.com/groups/393866897462725

About the Author

Shayne E Town is an author with a mission.
He once had a zest for life and was fuelled
by his passion for cooking as a chef for 13 years
before turning his hand to being a groundsman
where he was inspired by nature.

He had excellent health and a bright future, until life
threw him a curve ball and fibromyalgia took hold.
But Shayne is fighting back against the cruel and
debilitating illness, and his mission is to help others
and raise awareness for this misunderstood illness.

THE PAIN WE SUFFER IS REAL,
AND SO IS HOPE.

NEVER LOOK DOWN ON

PEOPLE WITH FIBROMYALGIA,

UNLESS YOU`RE THERE

TO HELP THEM GET BACK UP

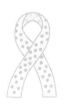

Notes

Notes

Notes

Notes

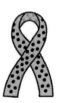

CPSIA information can be obtained at www.ICGtesting.com
Printed in the USA
BVOW02s1411010616

450344BV00007B/17/P